This book provides a concise, critical account of the mental health aspects of HIV infection as it affects patients, their partners and families, health professionals and other carers. The author, whose research, teaching and practice are conducted in an academic department of psychiatry, offers a considered and objective overview of the available information on psychological and behavioural aspects of AIDS and HIV, and challenges a number of ill-founded attitudes and opinions.

Prefaced by clear and up-to-date explanations of the biological and neurological effects of infection, the particular and often very complex problems encountered by patients and health workers are explored. Issues of fear and stigma are confronted, and many of the controversial issues in the psychiatry of AIDS, such as the impairment of cognitive function, are considered critically in an attempt to weigh up evidence and reach meaningful conclusions. Management options are discussed, and special attention is given to the needs of people growing up as homosexual in societies which explicitly approve a heterosexual lifestyle.

The author provides an informed assessment of reports and studies from around the world, including, where available, data from developing countries. He also contributes case histories, insights and practical advice which will commend this clear and thoughtful overview to a wide readership in the mental health field and beyond, including counsellors, psychotherapists, nurses, psychologists and psychiatrists.

This book provides a concise, detailed account of the mental health aspects of HIV infection as it affects patients, their partners and families, health professionals and other carers. The author, whose research, teaching and practice are conducted in an academic department of psychiatry, offers a considered and objective overview of the available information on psychological and behavioural aspects of AIDS and HIV, and challenges a number of ill-founded attitudes and opinions.

Prefaced by clear and up-to-date explanations of the biological and neurological effects of infection, the particular and often very complex problems encountered by patients and health workers are explored. Issues of fear and stigma are confronted, and many of the controversial issues in the psychiatry of AIDS, such as the impairment of cognitive function, are considered critically in an attempt to weigh up evidence and reach meaningful conclusions. Management options are discussed, and special attention is given to the needs of people growing up as homosexual in societies which explicitly approve a heterosexual lifestyle.

The author provides an informed assessment of reports and studies from around the world, including where available data from developing countries. He also contributes case histories, insights and practical advice which will commend this clear and meaningful overview to a wide readership in the mental health field and beyond, including counsellors, psychotherapists, nurses, psychologists and psychiatrists.

AIDS, HIV AND MENTAL HEALTH

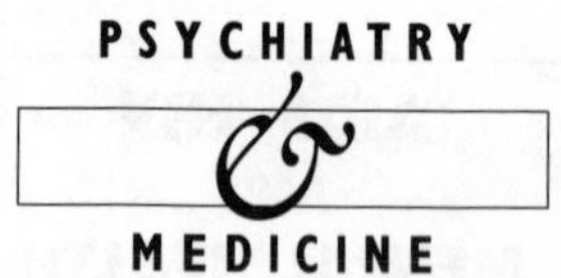

Over recent years, the extent of psychiatric morbidity among patients seen in general hospital practice and primary care has been well established. Physicians and surgeons are becoming increasingly aware of the importance of recognising and treating the psychiatric problems that their patients experience, and consultation–liaison psychiatry has become a distinct field for research and clinical practice. In the context of general medicine and its specialities, psychiatric morbidity may coexist with definite organic pathology or present largely with somatic symptoms in the absence of organic disease. This area is receiving more attention in postgraduate and undergraduate teaching, but there are few specialist textbooks which cover the topic.

This series is introduced to review particular areas of medicine in which psychological factors and psychiatric morbidity are especially significant. Each is written or edited by a clinician with extensive experience in the area, and combines clinical insight with a discussion of relevant research. The series is aimed at senior clinicians and trainees, particularly in psychiatry, internal medicine and general practice, and individual volumes will interest a wider audience in the health professions.

AIDS, HIV AND MENTAL HEALTH

MICHAEL B. KING

Academic Psychiatry,
Royal Free Hospital School of Medicine,
London, UK

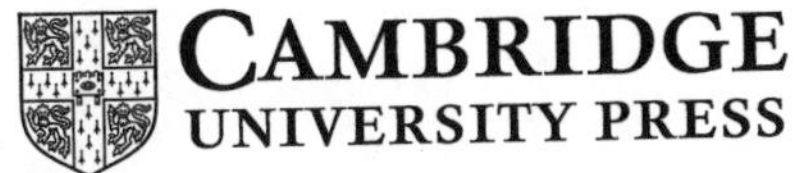

Published by the Press Syndicate of the University of Cambridge
The Pitt Building, Trumpington Street, Cambridge CB2 1RP
40 West 20th Street, New York, NY 10011-4211, USA
10 Stamford Road, Oakleigh, Melbourne 3166, Australia

First published 1993

Printed in Great Britain at the University Press, Cambridge

A catalogue record for this book is available from the British Library

Library of Congress cataloguing in publication data

King, Michael B.
AIDS, HIV and mental health/ Michael B. King.
p. cm.
Includes bibliographical references and index.
ISBN 0 521 42356 2 (pbk.)
1. AIDS (Disease) – Psychological aspects. 2. AIDS (Disease) – Patients – Mental health. 3. HIV infections – Psychological aspects. 4. AIDS phobia. I. Title
[DNLM: 1. Acquired Immunodeficiency Syndrome – psychology. 2. HIV Infections – psychology. WD 308 K53a 1993]
RC607.A26K55 1993
616.97′92′0019 – dc20
DNLM/DLC
for Library of Congress 92–48544 CIP

ISBN 0 521 45294 5 hardback
ISBN 0 521 42356 2 paperback

TAG

CONTENTS

PREFACE

As we reach the tenth anniversary of the discovery of the human immunodeficiency virus (HIV), much remains unclear about the nature of HIV infection and disease. The acquired immune deficiency syndrome (AIDS) has had major repercussions throughout Western and developing countries, no less in mental health than in other medical, social or political domains. The enormous developments which have occurred over these ten years have led to a confusing array of specialist information which, for the generalist, may be difficult to decipher or place in context. Thus, at the outset, it is important to stress what this book is *not* about. It is not a detailed review of every paper that has appeared on the psychiatry of AIDS. Nor does it contain extensive, technical accounts of the medical aspects of the illness which are better referred to in other sources. Nor does it pursue (too far) tempting side issues involving social or ethical aspects where they are not directly related to mental health. Nor is it primarily a guide to the psychiatric management of patients with AIDS. Rather, I have attempted to write a brief, critical account of the mental health aspects of HIV infection as it impacts on patients, professionals and other carers. Important evidence is reviewed, relating it to psychiatric clinical and research work in other fields and discussing practical management options. This is a 'put-in-context' book for those mental health professionals who wish to familiarise or update themselves with the relevant issues.

Goffman defined stigma as the 'situation of the individual who is disqualified from full social acceptance' (Goffman, 1968). Perhaps this theme more than any other underpins many of the mental health problems inherent to HIV infection. Only as AIDS, and the issues of sexuality and drug use which surround it, becomes more familiar and loses its fearful and negative associations, will people with HIV infection truly be free to confront their disorder.

Michael B. King
November 1992

Reference

Goffman E. (1968). *Stigma – Notes on the Management of Spoiled Identity* Harmondsworth, Penguin.

CHAPTER ONE

INTRODUCTION

AIDS was first recognised in homosexual men in the United States in 1980. Initially isolated from the serum of a haemophiliac patient in France by Montagnier in 1983, HIV is a retrovirus composed of RNA which can only replicate itself by invading host mammalian cells and by enlisting the cell machinery of that host. Since its discovery, our knowledge of the virus and its effects on the human body have expanded enormously. Only a brief account will be given here in order to introduce well-established information. Many points concerning the pathogenesis of HIV infection will be returned to in later chapters, but, for a full review of the scientific and medical aspects of the infection, the reader is recommended to consult an up-to-date text. Acquiring a detailed knowledge of HIV may not be necessary to understand many of the mental health sequelae of the infection. However, as will be stressed throughout this book, for those mental health professionals who work with HIV patients, a good knowledge is essential in order to maintain credibility with a patient group which is very well informed about the nature of the disease and new developments in the field.

Lymphocytes derived from thymus tissue, so-called T-cells, and a number of other cells in the body such as macrophages and microglial cells of the CNS, bear a genetic marker called CD4 which is an essential surface receptor for HIV to enter the cell. The portion of the CD4 receptor which is necessary for this process is called *soluble* CD4. The virus enters the body through breaks in mucous membranes after exchange of body fluids. It is now well known that exchange of semen or blood products form the commonest pattern of spread of the virus. Transmission may occur between people during unprotected, vaginal or anal sexual intercourse, during exchange of infected blood products, or from mother to child via the placenta or during parturition or breast feeding. Receptive anal intercourse is the activity which carries the highest risk of infection because of the increased likelihood of a breach occurring in the mucous membranes. Ordinary household contacts carry no risk.

Once HIV enters a host cell, it releases viral RNA which is converted into DNA by a process catalysed by the enzyme reverse transcriptase. In this way, copies of viral RNA can be produced. Viral DNA is subsequently integrated into the genome of the host cell where it remains dormant for long periods. Among the many genes making up the HIV, there are three which are well known and important; *gag* which codes for core proteins such as p24, *pol* which codes for the enzyme reverse transcriptase, and *env* which codes for viral envelope proteins like gp120.

Once the HIV has gained access to a new host it quickly spreads throughout the body. Between three and six months after transmission, antibodies to HIV become detectable in serum and, at this point, a so-called seroconversion illness, with symptoms similar to mild infectious mononucleosis, may occur. On occasion, seroconversion symptoms can be serious and significant immunosuppression occurs. A more severe seroconversion illness may be predictive of a shorter latent phase before appearance of HIV disease. Although antibodies may be effective at suppressing HIV in the early stages, it is unclear why the virus eventually eludes the immune response and becomes active. Clearly, a virus which attacks the immune system is in a class apart from other retroviruses. Further detail on the structure and functioning of the immune system is given in Chapter 11 in a consideration of psychological factors and immunity.

The mechanism of dormancy or what triggers the virus to reactivate and multiply itself within the cell is not fully understood. Co-factors in the development of impaired immunity and virus activation are likely to be very important. These include other viruses such as cytomegalovirus infection (CMV) or herpes viruses, but may also include less specific factors such as substance abuse or psychological distress. It has been postulated that emotional stress may act as a co-factor, making progression to active disease more likely. Nevertheless, over the years there is a slow, but cumulative, decline in CD4 lymphocytes with a subsequent imbalance of helper/suppressor ratios (CD4/CD8) in the immune system.

There are at least two forms of the virus, HIV-1 and HIV-2. It appears that HIV-2 also appeared in Africa and its rate of spread has been much less extensive. At the time of writing, there has been little impact of HIV-2 infection in most non-African countries. Unless otherwise stated, throughout this book HIV refers to HIV-1. The infection is classified according to the Centers for Disease Control (CDC 1987) into four principal stages or groups (table). Acute infection is classified as group I which may be

Table 1.1. *Classification according to the Centers for Disease Control (1987)*

Group I	**Acute infection (seroconversion)** – may occur up to three months after contact – usually asymptomatic but may have acute illness similar to infectious mononucleosis or more rarely encephalopathy and/or myelopathy
Group II	**Asymptomatic infection** – seropositive for HIV antibodies
Group III	**Persistent generalised lymphadenopathy (PGL)** – nodes at least 1 cm in diameter in two or more non-contiguous extrainguinal sites for at least three months – no history of opportunistic infections or persistent constitutional symptoms
Group IV	
Subgroup A	Constitutional disease (AIDS-related complex) – fever, weight loss, fatigue, night sweats
Subgroup B	Neurological disease – dementia, encephalitis, meningitis, peripheral neuropathy
Subgroup C	Secondary infectious disease
Subgroup D	Secondary cancers
Subgroup E	Other conditions

symptomless or, more rarely, presents as a severe illness with measurable immunosuppression. Group II consists of a latent period, in which there are no symptoms or signs, but people are none the less infectious. In group III there is development of persistent lymphadenopathy at two or more extrainguinal sites, an evolution which often goes undetected by the patient. Group IV includes a collection of subcategories in which more generalised symptoms are present, ranging from constitutional malaise with fever and weight loss to pneumonias, cancers and neurological disease.

Secondary diseases such as malignancies and opportunistic infections are much more likely to supervene when CD4 counts decline below 200 per μl. At this point, or in some cases earlier, the decision is taken to institute prophylactic treatments. For this reason, among others, from the 1st of January 1993 the Centers for Disease Control in the United States have adopted a major revision to the case definition. All HIV infected adolescents and adults without an AIDS indicator under the earlier classification, but who have a CD4 lymphocyte count of less than 200 per μl (or CD4 percentage less than 14) will be defined as having AIDS. In addition, recurrent pneumonia within a 12 month period, pulmonary tuberculosis and invasive cervical carcinoma in HIV infected persons have been added to the list of AIDS indicator conditions. The widened case definition will immediately increase the numbers of people with AIDS diagnosis. However, its utility in developing countries where immunological testing is less accessible remains in doubt. Moreover, CD4 counts are known to vary widely and hence an AIDS diagnosis made on one low count may be unnecessary and psychologically damaging. The World Health Organisation European Centre for the epidemiological monitoring of AIDS based in Paris recommends that a common European definition, to include the three extra indicator diseases, be adopted but has rejected the extension of the definition of AIDS on the basis of CD4 counts alone (Ancelle-Park, 1993).

Evidence from cohort studies, both in the United States and Europe, indicates that up to 60 per cent of seropositive individuals will develop symptoms of HIV disease within 12 years (Lifson et al., 1990). Careful analysis of cohort studies also reveals that age is an important factor in progression, with younger patients surviving longer from transmission (Lee et al., 1991) It must be remembered, however, that, since HIV was implicated as the causative agent leading to AIDS, treatments have changed enormously and prognosis for newly infected people may be much better. There is good evidence that use of zidovudine (formerly called azidothymidine or AZT), inhaled pentamidine, other prophylactic antimicrobial compounds and antiviral agents, particularly against cytomegalovirus infection (CMV), is having a significant effect on reducing morbidity and progression to AIDS.

The epidemiology of AIDS continues to change. Three waves or patterns of infection throughout the world have been described. It would appear that the virus arose in Africa through successive mutations from earlier, possibly simian forms (McClure & Schulz, 1989). Up to 30 per cent of men and women in the sexually active populations of some African countries may be HIV seropositive. Spread to the West occurred in the 1960s and 1970s, principally via homosexual men. Homosexual men and intravenous drug users in Western countries have formed what is referred to as the second wave of the epidemic. The third wave of infection is that currently occurring in the more socially deprived parts of USA and Europe and in the developing countries in South East Asia, South America and the Caribbean where spread is linked to a complicated mix of drug use and both homosexual and heterosexual spread. Each new twist in the epidemic brings new medical, psychological and social problems.

CHAPTER TWO

FEAR OF INFECTION AND PSYCHOLOGICAL REACTION TO THE DIAGNOSIS

It barely needs stating that AIDS evokes widespread fear in many people. For some, however, this fear may reach obsessional proportions quite beyond that expected in the normal course of events. In this chapter, the issue of fear of AIDS in people who are not known to be seropositive will be addressed, as well as other related syndromes in seronegative individuals and the types of emotional reactions which occur in response to HIV antibody testing.

Fear of HIV infection

People with varying degrees of concern that they may have contracted HIV are often characterised as the 'worried well'. This term has been applied so widely that it can include any person who perceives him or herself to have been at risk of AIDS, continues to worry after the exclusion of infection by medical examination, is compulsively and obsessionally fearful, repeatedly importunes for medical help despite adequate reassurance or is delusionally convinced of harbouring the virus (Miller, Acton & Hedge, 1988, Faulstich, 1987, Bor et al., 1989, Davey & Green, 1991). Other labels, such as 'AIDS phobia', 'AIDS panic' and 'pseudo-AIDS' have also been applied in similar contexts (Hausman, 1983, Jacob et al., 1987, Miller et al., 1985). None is helpful as fear of the infection presents differently depending on the objective degree and type of risk as well as the personality, background and previous psychiatric history of the person.

Normal concerns about risk of infection

Many patients who become fearful of HIV infection are not seen by AIDS physicians, venereologists, psychologists, or counsellors. They consult their family doctor. Primary health care is the resource with which most patients fearful of contracting AIDS make first contact (King, 1989*a*). Many may be reluctant, at least initially, to consult services for sexually transmitted diseases or an HIV clinic. Some will be reassured by advice about the infection while others may require the evidence of a negative test. Although it has been suggested that this group of people be described as having 'AIDS anxiety' (Miller et al., 1988), the term contributes nothing to the understanding of such fears. Many people at different periods of their lives dread the possibility of contracting a serious illness such as cancer or coronary disease (Baur, 1988). There is no evidence to suggest that people who have brief periods of anxiety about AIDS are distinctive from these other groups in any important way. Many of those who become anxious about AIDS may have put themselves at a significant degree of risk through unprotected penetrative sex or use of IV drugs. The majority do not enter a state of chronic anxiety about the possibility of infection. None the less, media campaigns may spark off anxiety in a section of the population who would not otherwise have been concerned (Lewin & Williams, 1988). For example, such campaigns in Great Britain led to major increases in demand for HIV testing with no increase in the proportion testing seropositive (Beck et al., 1990).

Persistent fears of infection

People who are not reassured by objective review of their likelihood of exposure, physical examination or HIV antibody testing may become chronically disturbed. They may become persuaded that symptoms which are related to physical manifestations of anxiety or depression are indicative of HIV disease. These include insomnia, excessive sweating, reduced appetite with weight loss, looseness of the bowels, reduced concentration and forgetfulness, anxiety-induced cough and breathlessness. They may become preoccupied with normal bodily processes with which they had been previously unaware, for example, by focusing on minor skin blemishes or normal lymph node hypertrophy or becoming preoccupied with ordinary hair loss. Their daily lives develop into a repetitive routine of bodily checking which, although providing brief reassurance, eventually leads to an escalation of concern. Elaborate rituals of washing and decontamination may be indistinguishable from those observed in patients with other obsessive–compulsive syndromes related to cleanliness. Exhausted, their thoughts become fixed on the likelihood of physical decline, suffering and death and many acquire elaborate rituals to avoid contaminating others. Seeking constant reassurance from friends or family, they become unable to enjoy even the most basic of daily pleasures. Depressive thoughts include the inevitability of decline and death, guilt over past behaviours and fear that they may have contaminated others. Up to half may become acutely depressed and suicidal (Miller et al., 1988). In an account of eight cases of patients with unfounded fear of AIDS treated at a university hospital in Finland, it was reported that three of the patients committed suicide and one of them had overt suicidal tendencies (Vuorio, Aarela & Lehtinen, 1990).

Many consult their family doctor. Fifty-three per-cent of a sample of 270 London general practitioners, interviewed about their involvement with HIV issues, reported patients who consulted them with recurrent fears about contracting AIDS (King, 1989*a*). Three-quarters of patients who consulted repeatedly for worries about possible HIV infection were male and only two were known to be seropositive. The doctors attempted to counsel and educate the patients and only resorted to referral to mental health services in 20 cases.

Persistent anxiety about unsubstantiated HIV infection is often associated with previous fears of illness, particularly venereal disease. Health professionals working in services for sexually transmitted diseases are familiar with patients who become excessively concerned about a wide range of 'symptoms' which suggest venereal infection. Between 30 and 40 per-cent of attenders at STD clinics may have significant psychiatric problems (Pedder & Goldberg, 1970, Catalan et al., 1981, Ikkos et al., 1987, Barczak et al., 1988). Besides general psychological distress, difficulties are encountered in the context of the service, such as psychosomatic complaints focused on the genitalia (Woodward, 1981), general hypochondriasis (Ross, 1987) and venereophobia (Oates & Gomez, 1984). Those patients with specific illness fears frequently misinterpret physical symptoms and are left unreassured by the explanations of clinic staff. They may become importuning and depressed (Frost, 1985).

Uncontrolled studies of people with persistent fears of HIV infection suggest that they are more likely to be concerned about issues of sexuality (Miller et al., 1988) and guilt (Davey & Green, 1991). They may be unable to reconcile homosexual impulses or develop and sustain either heterosexual or homosexual relationships. Their families of origin may have been too restrictive in moral or religious terms and unable to tolerate adult expression of sexuality. Occasional reports of the appearance of fear of AIDS in early adolescence at the time of maximal sexual change and development have also been published (Lewin & Williams, 1988). A history of psychiatric disorder or personality problems is common. Patients are often introverted, prone to anxiety, and reveal a history of previous concern about health (Todd, 1989). They are also more likely to have partners or close friends who have HIV infection or AIDS.

Treatment approaches have applied principally cognitive–behavioural techniques, with or without antidepressant therapy, in similar style to those already well established for treatment of obsessive–compulsive disorders. Miller et al. (1988) have described a model of treatment based on the two principal characteristics of hypochondriacal syndromes, namely preoccupation with bodily health and the seeking of reassurance. Reassurance is sought as a means of avoidance of the fear of illness, but leads inevitably to an exacerbation of the anxiety in a manner analogous to that in which compulsive rituals aggravate fear of contamination. Principal goals of treatment are to enable patients to reinterpret body sensations as physiological expressions of anxiety rather than as indications of infection, and to challenge the cascading nature of negative, anxious thoughts about possible infection. At the same time, an agreement is made with the patient that reassurance on the likelihood of HIV infection will not be given. It is crucial that patients understand the theoretical background to these interventions and that their rationale is clear. It may be helpful for patients to reframe the problem as *fear* of AIDS rather than AIDS itself, to seek to assuage guilt, possibly by confession, and to avoid taking an interest in information on AIDS on the presumption that such information is only of salience to those actually infected (Davey & Green, 1991).

Mr T. was a 36 year old heterosexual who drove a London taxi. He was happily married with two young sons and was in excellent physical health. He repeatedly attended health service and private STD clinics, with a conviction that he had become infected with HIV, but was only briefly reassured by negative test results. This concern did not appear to be provoked by a sexual liaison outside his marriage, or by any ambivalence about his sexual orientation. Years before his presentation he had become convinced that he had contracted gonorrhoea during which time he experienced vague discomfort in his penis and testicles and ruminated about passing the infection to his wife. Although he had no personal history of psychiatric disorder, his sister was reported to suffer similar fears of illness. He ruminated on every bodily symptom that might be suggestive of the development of the disorder.

He attended for repeated HIV testing, always using a false name and address. Eventually, he became convinced that he might contract HIV from the test procedure itself, and would go to elaborate lengths to ensure that doctors or nurses taking the blood sample followed his instructions. Becoming acutely depressed, he discovered that he could not maintain his employment. After painstaking interpretation of the link between physical expression of anxiety and the symptoms he was experiencing, he was started on a course of antidepressants. He panicked when he developed excessive sweating, but, after explanation that this was a side effect of the drug, complied with the treatment. Concurrently, he underwent a course of cognitive–behavioural therapy, the aim of which was to enable him to challenge his faulty thinking and test out the objective evidence for infection. The agreement in therapy was to avoid discussing AIDS and all reassurance was withdrawn. Six months later, although left with some residual concern about the possibility of infection, his depression had lifted, and he was able to resume driving. One year later, he had sustained this improvement and was capable of enlisting cognitive techniques to avoid the escalation of anxiety.

In a small uncontrolled trial of treatment of this type Miller et al. (1988) reported considerable success. Salt, Miller & Perry (1989) also reported early experience with paradoxical techniques in which the patient was instructed to continue to worry about the possibility of infection. Patients recording and subsequently playing back their ruminations has been recommended for the treatment of obsessive–compulsive disorders (Stern & Drummond, 1991) and may also be worth undertaking, although, in my experience, this is not popular with patients. Occasionally, this syndrome of excessive fear of HIV infection may be one part of a major depression which recovers after standard treatment with antidepressant drugs (Jenike & Pato, 1986). Unfortunately, not all patients with this constellation of symptoms do well, and they can take up considerable amounts of clinical time.

Delusional conviction of HIV infection

Delusional conviction of HIV infection occupies an extreme position on the spectrum of AIDS concern. Patients are resolutely convinced that they are infected, and will often act on this explicit assumption. Negative antibody tests have no reassuring effect and are usually not sought, as the patient regards any objective confirmation of his or her illness as unnecessary. Mahorney & Cavenar (1988) described three cases of delusional conviction of AIDS in patients with psychotic depression, none of whom had a history which would have placed them at risk for the infection. Guilty delusions of venereal infection have long been known to be an accompaniment of psychotic depression in some people and these authors regarded the appearance of a delusional conviction of AIDS as a contemporary theme in patients 'whose sense of guilt seeks a rational and tangible form'. All three patients completely lost their delusions about AIDS after standard treatment of their depression. There seems to be nothing particularly unique about this syndrome. Delusional conviction of AIDS or HIV infection may simply be a contemporary expression of psychotic illness which has little to do with actual risk status or previous concern about the infection.

Other psychological syndromes in seronegative people

Factitious HIV infection

Rarely, patients may falsely claim that they are HIV antibody positive, in my own experience, this is usually in order to secure social support or financial assistance. In some countries, support, particularly the provision of housing, for people with HIV infection, is relatively generous. Alternatively, drug users may occasionally pretend to have HIV infection to ensure a supply of maintenance medication and forestall any attempt on the part of drug service personnel to encourage abstinence. It is normal practice in AIDS units to retest all unknown patients who appear to require treatment, with the important proviso that a negative antibody test calls for antigen testing before assuming that the patient is malingering.

There are rare reports of patients who masquerade as HIV antibody positive for a variety of psychopathological reasons. It may be difficult to be confident that such presentations are not based on hypochondriacal conviction and an attendant denial of seronegative status (Wu, Kennedy & Paradise, 1988), but some are a variant of Munchausen's syndrome in which the patient is admitted with a dramatic illness and is later discovered to have fabricated the whole presentation (Kavalier, 1989). When the syndrome occurs in drug users who are already emaciated and in poor health as a result of their drug use, detection of the syndrome can take some time (Zuger & O'Dowd, 1992). Munchausen's syndrome is a rare disorder in which people importune for medical help by falsely adopting florid, usually acute syndromes (Asher, 1951). Their presentations are often regarded as medical emergencies which lead to repeated medical and surgical interventions. Eventually, the distinction between genuine and factitious disorder may become difficult as patients suffer the complications of repeated, unnecessary surgery. Those patients who masquerade with psychological disorders are even rarer. Psychopathological mechanisms underlying the syndrome are poorly understood, but there is a fundamental difference between the compulsive, dramatic presentations of Munchausen's syndrome and minor degrees of abnormal illness behaviour in order to avoid ordinary responsibilities. There is little evidence that cases of Munchausen AIDS are in any fundamental way different to other presentations of the syndrome.

• *Deliberate attempts to contract HIV*

There have now been several reports of individuals who appear to have deliberately placed themselves at high risk for contracting the virus. Frances, Wilkstrom and Alcena (1985) reported on a homosexual man, who, after several failed suicide attempts, put himself repeatedly, and apparently intentionally, at risk through unsafe sexual contacts. While it was not clear from the report whether the man contracted the virus by way of these efforts, he did eventually develop AIDS. This type of behaviour may be an overt expression of other more common parasuicidal actions such as dangerous driving and drinking that are daily phenomena in our society. No doubt, variations also occur in the world of drug dependence, but most are unlikely to come to the attention of doctors or psychologists.

Psychological reactions to testing

Concern about psychological reactions to HIV antibody testing has long been a serious consideration in whether testing should be performed at all. Particularly in the early years after testing became widely available, accepted wisdom held that there was little to gain from routine testing. Giving people knowledge of their serostatus when there was little that could be done to prevent or forestall the development of HIV disease was considered unnecessary and possibly detrimental to their psychological health. The argument that awareness of serostatus was necessary to protect partners and prevent spread of the virus was countered by the view that people should, in any case, adopt the precautions recommended to prevent transmission. In short, if in doubt presume seropositivity. This argument held sway despite the likelihood that many people who needlessly worried about HIV infection might have been fundamentally reassured by a test. In addition, despite suggestions that suicide was a possible consequence for people learning of their diagnosis (Glass, 1988), there was little systematic evidence that testing threatened psychological health.

Recently, Samuel Perry and his team in New York have published a series of papers (Perry et al., 1990*a*,*b*,*c*) concerning emotional distress at the time of testing, responses to testing and the relationship with previous psychiatric disorder. Through advertising and contacts with medical clinics 218 volunteers were recruited. All were physically well and unaware of their antibody status. Emotional state was assessed by use of standardised, psychological questionnaires and by visual analogue scales at enlistment two weeks before notification of the test result, immediately prior to, and after, notification and subsequently at two and ten weeks after notification. Subjects were also assessed by structured psychiatric interview at entry to the study to determine lifetime rates of psychiatric disorder. All assessments were completed by 174 men and 44 women.

Not unexpectedly, there were high rates of distress just prior to notification which fell most quickly in those people who were subsequently found to be HIV negative. Reported relief was immediate and sustained for those who received a negative result and, as over 90 per cent of all patients tested in clinics are seronegative, these findings provided strong evidence for the power of a negative test to ease unnecessary worry about the possibility of HIV infection.

Patients who tested HIV antibody positive also showed a decrease in psychiatric distress from levels at entry, no doubt reflecting high baseline levels in people who are about to undergo antibody testing. Those seropositive subjects who had incorrectly predicted that they would have a negative test were no more likely to suffer psychological distress on notification of the positive result than those who already suspected that they were positive. Furthermore, the scores of seropositive individuals ten weeks after notification were significantly lower than at entry, demonstrating little long-term psychological damage from knowledge of their antibody status. This may have been due, at least in part, to the extensive pre- and post-test counselling which took place during the project. It may have also reflected the fact that fear and uncertainty about HIV serostatus may be harder to cope with in the long term than the definite knowledge of a positive result.

Suicidal ideas were investigated in the same cohort of volunteers (Perry et al., 1990*b*). Although suicidal ideation was present in up to one-third of people at the outset, this did not increase after HIV testing and two months later had dropped considerably, even among the seropositives. None the less, 15 per cent of subjects, regardless of subsequent serostatus, continued to report at least fleeting suicidal ideas at the ten week follow-up point. This finding may merely indicate the ubiquity of suicidal thoughts among people in the wider community, or it may have been a reflection of the psychiatric state of the population in the study. The latter explanation is likely to be the most valid. Structured psychiatric interviews at entry to the study revealed very high rates of current and lifetime disorder in this population. These volunteers reported a rate of *Diagnostic and Statistical Manual of Mental Disorders* of the American Psychiatric Association, 3rd edn. revised (DSMIIIR) Axis I disorders almost double that in comparable community groups in the United States (Robins et al., 1984). The high rates were striking even after controlling for substance abuse disorders. Lifetime rates for mood disorders were seven times that for age-matched community samples. Interestingly, there was a trend for more homosexual men in the sample, who were subsequently found to be seropositive, to report current or past psychiatric disorder.

There are several possible explanations for this finding. It might be that people at risk for HIV infection have higher rates of psychiatric disorder. The homosexual men who proved to be seropositive may at some level have realised that they were likely to be seropositive, and this premonition might have influenced their presentation. This second possibility is not borne out by the rating scale measurements, however, which did not differ between those seropositives who had predicted a positive test result and those who had not. It might be that high rates of psychiatric disorder in some way predispose people to behaviour that puts them at greater risk of infection. This is discussed in Chapter 3 on psychiatric associations of HIV infection. A further possibility is that volunteers who take part in studies such as this one have higher rates of disorder. They may be more concerned about health or with the possibility of HIV infection, or they may suffer emotional problems for which they hope to gain help in the study. In conclusion, it is important to emphasise that information about the psychopathology of asymptomatic adults who perceive themselves to be at risk of HIV infection are better established from epidemiological than from volunteer studies.

Further information on the effects of HIV antibody testing has come from data on the San Francisco General Hospital Cohort (Moulton et al., 1991). The impact of HIV antibody testing on 107 homosexual men in San Francisco was examined 12 months after notification. Knowledge of HIV antibody status reduced distress in persons who had incorrectly perceived themselves to be infected with HIV and did not appear to induce significant distress in those whose expectation of a positive result was confirmed. Both groups reported lower distress than men with Aids Related Complex (ARC) or AIDS, suggesting that distress was related more to symptomatology than to knowledge of antibody status. Thus, HIV testing may bring considerable benefits to seronegative subjects who believe themselves to be seropositive, and must be balanced against the more limited and temporary aggravation of distress in seropositives who receive confirmation of their test result expectation.

Although long-term effects seem to be minimal, there is no doubt that HIV testing is a harrowing experience for most people. What can be done to ameliorate this distress? It is obvious that patients should be counselled and closely supported throughout, and that the delay between testing and the provision of a result is minimal. There have been few attempts systematically to evaluate counselling, in part because of objections to randomising people to a 'no treatment' condition. In a study related to those just described, Perry et al. (1991) attempted to delineate the effective elements of counselling at the time of HIV antibody testing. Volunteers were randomised to one of three intervention groups: counselling, counselling plus a three-session educational interactive video programme about HIV and counselling together with six individual sessions of stress prevention training. This latter training employed cognitive–behavioural methods to enhance self-control, challenge dysfunctional thoughts and assumptions, to problem solve and increase assertiveness. No major differences were found between the three interventions for patients who subsequently tested seronegative. For those with a positive test result, however, stress prevention training showed significant benefits over the two other interventions in reducing stress. Unfortunately, follow-up of people taking part was limited to three months. As already discussed, a control group of subjects who received no counselling was not included, as it was considered unethical by the researchers. It is a peculiar feature of the AIDS field that counselling has become so sacrosanct, that controlled trials to assess its efficacy are not considered ethical if they include a group who do not receive it. Bad news of many types is given without counselling in medical and other fields, and, although it is not in any way suggested that this is a good thing, it does indicate that counselling is not yet universally considered essential. It may well be that counselling services which have developed in the AIDS field are an important model for other areas of medicine, but, without definite demonstration of their efficacy, expansion to other services will be patchy and dependent on local enthusiasm.

Conclusions

HIV disease presents in varied and subtle ways, frequently mimicking other medical conditions. Patients who are fearful of having contracted the virus may misinterpret normal bodily function or the physical manifestations of anxiety and depression as symptoms of HIV disease. They may become obsessively concerned with minor bodily changes, the fear growing to dominate their thinking and interfere with concentration. There is often a history of fear of other illnesses, particularly sexually transmitted diseases.

Surveys in primary medical care would suggest that, although fear of AIDS is not uncommon in the general population, extreme concern is much less common. Although there is little to suggest that the psychopathology of fear of HIV is markedly different from other hypochondriacal syndromes, attendant issues of stigmatisation, sexuality, past sexual behaviour, and use of drugs places special pressures on sufferers. Unless these aspects of HIV are fully considered, patients' fears may not be handled appropriately. Although the risk of suicide is small, it is real and may be associated with past psychiatric disorder. Intervention of a cognitive–behavioural type appears to be most successful. A contract is established with the patient within which thoughts and assumptions are examined and challenged while reassurance is withheld. Antidepressant medication may be a necessary adjunct in cases where depressed mood is a major part of the presentation and more particularly where depression is the primary problem. Rarely, the conviction of disease may take on delusional proportions when there appears to be no logical connection between the conviction and past risk behaviours. Here, traditional methods of treatment are indicated.

It is now clear that, although HIV antibody testing provokes considerable apprehension for most who undergo it, emotional distress is soon relieved, regardless of the test result. For patients who are HIV antibody positive, a cognitive–behavioural programme may achieve further reduction of stress. Much more work is needed to establish the efficacy of counselling for HIV infection.

CHAPTER THREE

PERSISTING PSYCHOLOGICAL DISORDER

It is clear that HIV provokes considerable anxiety and that antibody testing is a particular stress. It is also clear, however, that the majority of people found to be HIV antibody positive on testing make adjustments to their diagnosis. In this chapter the nature and prevalence of persisting psychological disorders in people with HIV infection and AIDS, and the effect of such disorders on progression of the infection, will be considered.

Psychiatric referrals of patients with HIV infection

Early in the AIDS pandemic in the USA, high levels of psychiatric distress were reported in people with AIDS. One of the earliest attempts to establish the prevalence of psychiatric disorder among inpatients was by Perry and Tross (1984) in which the medical notes of 51 men and one woman admitted with AIDS were surveyed at the New York Hospital. Psychiatric complications recorded anywhere in the notes, as well as the use of psychiatric consultations, were assessed. Eighty-three per cent of patients were said to show mood disturbance and 65 per cent organic mental syndromes. Despite this high rate of morbidity, psychiatric consultation was requested for only ten patients of whom only one was given a psychiatric diagnosis at discharge. Psychiatric consultation was sought most commonly for behavioural management, diagnostic assessment or because patients requested it. All but one of the patients were white, middle-class homosexual men. While at first sight these are very high levels of psychiatric need, the study was limited by the method of data collection. In common with many early studies, no comparison group was included. Assessments were made directly from the records by raters with a psychological training who judged the content of the entries on face value. Thus, assessments, either of diagnosis or therapeutic interventions, may have been biased. For example, not all interventions, particularly those of an informal, empathic nature, so frequently provided by a range of medical and non-medical staff, are entered in the records. Nevertheless, on the basis of their findings, the authors recommended more systematic monitoring of patients for functional and organic mental syndromes and the provision of appropriate after-care.

Another early report of the nature of distress in patients referred for psychiatric help was that by Dilley et al. (1985). Of 40 patients with AIDS admitted to San Francisco General Hospital over a nine-month period, 13 required psychiatric consultation. Depression was the commonest reason given by physicians for referral. Principal problems reported in this study have been echoed in many subsequent series of patients with HIV infection referred for psychiatric consultation. There is uncertainty about the nature and progression of the illness, misgivings about treatments, feelings of social isolation and abandonment, and beliefs that AIDS is a form of retribution for past behaviour. Reactions to HIV and AIDS were essentially similar to responses to other life-threatening illnesses. There was numbness, anger and fears of disability, pain, disfiguration and death and loss of future opportunities, health, liberty and treasured relationships. The patients in the study were gay or bisexual, mainly white and middle-class men, who lived alone. Although reflecting the profile of patients with AIDS in San Francisco at that time, case series such as this also contain inherent biases as to patient profile and local availability of services.

There have been several other reported case series of patients seen for psychiatric consultation in hospital or as ambulatory outpatients. In an Australian study, it was reported that 22 (15 per cent) of 150 patients with AIDS admitted to a Sydney hospital between February 1985 and May 1986 were referred for psychiatric consultation (Buhrich & Cooper, 1987). All were young, homosexual men. There were a wide variety of presentations, with ten suffering organic brain syndromes, five with psychoses which were possibly of organic origin, and five with mood disorders. The authors noted that the ward milieu was sensitive to possible emotional problems, particularly to adjustment reactions, and hence only major psychiatric issues or management difficulties triggered a referral.

In a similar study, this time in the Netherlands, of 270 inpatients with

HIV infection, 51 (19 per cent) were referred for psychiatric assessment (Sno et al., 1989). Of the 40 referrals with AIDS, all were homosexual or bisexual men reflecting the predominance of this group among AIDS cases in that country at the time. Commonest reasons for referral were for counselling, evaluation of depression and treatment of delirium. Very low rates of suicidal inclination among patients were reported. There was an upswing in referral during the period of the study which the authors attributed to the opening of the specialist unit and the participation of a psychiatrist at weekly meetings of the AIDS treatment team.

In a retrospective case note survey of 60 patients admitted over a 30-month period to a specialised inpatient facility in San Francisco for HIV infected people with psychological problems, depression, dementia and psychosis were the leading diagnoses (Baer, 1989). In contrast to some reports and perhaps reflecting reasons for admission, all but one had experienced suicidal impulses before entry to the unit. The most common stressors in patients with adjustment disorders were newly diagnosed HIV-related symptoms, perception of progression of disease, loss of a love relationship or a social crisis. Although dementia syndromes were recognised, results of laboratory and radiographic studies were not always consistent. A team of staff provided counselling, patient advocacy, and help with financial and emotional concerns outside hospital. Patients with dementia presented particular problems of increased dependency or disinhibited behaviour and displayed unusual sensitivity to adverse effects of antipsychotic medication. The study was limited to case note data which was scrutinised in a completely open fashion by the psychiatrist in charge. None the less, it provides a useful insight to management of patients with HIV infection who require admission for major psychiatric problems.

It is immediately clear from these reports that findings vary enormously depending upon the nature and location of the AIDS service. Two recent reports further reveal the difficulties of generalising from findings such as these. In a study of 324 self-referrals over a three-year period to an outpatient psychiatric clinic specialising in the treatment of HIV-related problems, O'Dowd et al. (1991) reported that adjustment disorder was the most common diagnosis. One-third to one-half of patients were assigned a diagnosis of substance abuse. Major affective disorders were uncommon and patients with ARC were no more likely to suffer a diagnosis of adjustment or depressive disorder than those in other HIV subgroups, a point which will be returned to in a later part of this chapter. Conversely, Seth et al. (1991), in describing a case series of 60 referrals made to a psychiatric team liaising with an AIDS service in central London, noted that affective disorders were much more common than adjustment disorders. This inconsistency does not necessarily reflect varying diagnostic habits. The difference lies in the types of patients seen in each service. In the first, the population served by the clinic was distinct from those in many earlier reports in consisting of mainly black and Spanish-speaking patients, just over half of whom were women. Intravenous drug use and heterosexual intercourse were the commonest modes of HIV transmission. Forty-four per cent had had previous psychiatric treatment. Despite self-referral, a high incidence of non-appearance for first appointments or subsequent drop-out persisted, despite the efforts of the staff. Patients most likely to return for further help were those on drug maintenance programmes or those given other prescriptions. Thus, this service reflected the chaotic background of many patients who were infected by, or at risk for, HIV in that particular area of New York. Seth et al. (1991) commented that most patients with adjustment disorders in their service were seen by counsellors and psychologists rather than by psychiatrists.

The principal limitation of these reports is a failure to make a comparison with referrals to psychiatry from other medical teams. It is impossible to place AIDS referrals in context without information on the pattern of referrals from other medical services. In one recent study, however, a controlled comparison of referrals was conducted (Ellis, Collis & King, 1993). Seventy patients with HIV infection referred to the liaison psychiatry service of a London teaching hospital were compared with 70 age and sex-matched controls referred for psychiatric assessment from general medical and surgical services in the same hospital. Organic, adjustment, mood and personality disorders were the most common primary diagnoses. The prevalence of these disorders did not differ significantly between HIV and control groups except in the case of alcohol dependence which was commoner among the controls. Forty-four per cent of the HIV group and 30 per cent of the controls fulfilled DSMIIIR criteria for a secondary diagnosis of non-alcohol psychoactive drug abuse. A history of psychiatric problems was more common in the control group. There was little difference in management between the two groups with numbers of patients requiring day-patient and out-patient treatment being almost identical in HIV and control groups. These results demonstrate that, in an appropriately controlled comparison, there was little difference in the form of psychological disorder between patients with AIDS and patients with other medical problems who are referred to psychiatry. While the content of problems differed, arrangements for patients were essentially similar. Contrary to other reports, a history of psychiatric disorder was more common in the controls than in the HIV group. Uncontrolled reports were helpful in first delineating the types of psychiatric problems in people with HIV referred to psychiatrists, but, in order to develop services further, we now require further data that are meaningful in the context of other services.

Prevalence of psychiatric disorder

Although reports of case series referred to psychiatrists provide an important insight into the types of disorders referred, and the management employed to deal with them, they cannot indicate the incidence, prevalence or relative importance of each type of psychiatric problem encountered in HIV infection. To do this, it is necessary to apply epidemiological methods to the study of unselected groups of patients, preferably utilising comparison groups of people without infection and employing a prospective design.

Selecting appropriate patients and controls, however, is fraught with difficulty. Enlisting an unselected group of patients with HIV infection is impossible, short of conducting an intrusive, house-to-house survey which would, in any case, be unacceptable on ethical grounds. Samples of convenience are therefore often used, be they hospital admissions, clinic attenders, responders to advertisement or members of support groups in the community. None is completely satisfactory from a strictly methodological point of view. Avoiding bias in the selection of comparison subjects is also difficult. Homosexual, seronegative controls are an obvious choice in studies of seropositive, homosexual men, but enlisting such controls is difficult. So-called representative samples of gay men in the community are difficult to enlist, if indeed, they exist. Seronegative controls, selected from among attenders to clinics for sexually transmitted diseases, or from among patients who have recently received a negative HIV antibody test, are subject to particular biases. The former are likely to be more sexually active and may be subject to higher rates of psychiatric disorder (Ikkos et al., 1987, Barczak et al., 1988) The latter, after having just received a negative test, will not be in their usual mental state and, if participation is postponed, their show rate at a later date purely for the purposes of research is unlikely to be high. Heterosexuals are unsuitable for controlled studies in which gay men predominate. Young people with other serious illnesses are not easy to recruit in sufficient numbers and again it is difficult to control for sexuality.

Comparison groups of seronegative drug users are usually chosen from among service attenders but again they may not be representative of all drug users.

In the study of any disorder, a longitudinal design provides the most powerful estimates of incidence and risk factors for physical or psychiatric complications. However, prospective studies are expensive and time consuming to mount, and depend upon minimising numbers of drop-outs.

Although such difficulties are complex, a variety of methods has been elaborated to circumvent them. Cross-sectional studies cannot provide information on risk factors, but they do afford valuable snapshots of a disorder, particularly when there is an urgent need for information. While not the most satisfactory alternative, uncontrolled studies may be conducted, using standardised psychiatric rating scales or structured interviews, the results of which can be contrasted directly with data obtained using the same instruments in other, analogous settings. Case-control studies may provide information on possible risk factors, and thus avoid the requirement for long-term follow-ups, but are subject to crucial biases in the selection of cases or controls. Some of the more important work in the field is described below in an attempt to draw out conclusions on the pattern of psychiatric disturbance in HIV infection.

Cross sectional studies

In one of the earliest controlled assessments of psychiatric disorder in patients with HIV infection, which had considerable influence at the time, it was claimed that homosexual men with or without HIV infection suffered considerably higher rates of lifetime psychiatric disorder than heterosexual controls (Atkinson et al., 1988). Fifteen homosexual men with AIDS, 13 with AIDS-related symptoms, 17 who were mildly symptomatic or asymptomatic, and 11 seronegative were compared with 22 heterosexual controls. A lifetime history of at least one psychiatric disorder was noted among 80 per cent of men with AIDS, 84.6 per cent of those with ARC, 88.2 per cent of those with few or no symptoms and 100 per cent of seronegatives. In contrast only 59 per cent of heterosexual men recorded such a diagnosis. Diagnoses were principally anxiety, depression and substance abuse. A high rate of neuropsychological impairment was also found in these patients which is further discussed in Chapter 5 on the neuropsychiatry of HIV infection. There were major problems with this study which, despite its public impact at the time, greatly limited the conclusions. Subjects were volunteers in a longitudinal health study, numbers were very small and selection bias of both subjects and controls was very likely. The authors also took little cognisance of the considerable criticism that has been made of the accuracy and validity of lifetime diagnosis (Parker, 1987).

In contrast, in other work around the world, low rates of current disorder have been reported for people with HIV infection. In a survey of attenders with HIV infection to two surveillance clinics in London, I carried out a standardised assessment of the current and past psychiatric state of 192 people with HIV infection, to estimate prevalence of psychiatric disorder (King, 1989*a*). Patients were unselected, consecutive attenders who were not seeking psychiatric help. Bias was inevitable, however, in that more patients with AIDS and HIV related symptoms were included than was predicted, no doubt because symptoms provoked unscheduled or more frequent visits to the clinic. Most were homosexual or bisexual men which reflected the pattern of HIV infection in London at the time. The prevalence of psychiatric disorder in this population was 33 per cent. Diagnoses made in accordance with the 9th edition of the *International Classification of Diseases* (*ICD9*) were mainly anxiety states, neurotic depression and prolonged adjustment disorders. Predictors of a current psychiatric diagnosis were past emotional problems, psychiatric treatment or obsessive concern about minor symptoms. Although 29 per cent of patients had been the recipients of open hostility from others concerning their diagnosis and 25 per cent of the gay men had been discriminated against on the basis of their sexuality, there were no links between such experiences and psychiatric disorder (King, 1989*b*). Although the prevalence of psychiatric disorder was lower than in earlier studies, it was remarkably similar to other populations of people presenting with serious physical disorder with whom the same structured psychiatric interview had been used. It was concluded that, although there were particular difficulties for people with HIV infection, principally relating to the stigma of the infection, rates of psychiatric problems were comparable to those in populations with other serious illnesses, and were not particularly linked to discrimination. Conclusions were limited, however, in that the population studied were predominantly middle-class, white, gay men who were socially stable and adept at using the health service to their best advantage.

In a further study of cross-sectional associations with psychiatric disorder in homosexual or bisexual men, Ostrow et al. (1989) also demonstrated that *perceived* HIV-related symptoms, such as lymphadenopathy, weight loss and fever, were related to higher scores on psychological rating scales regardless of HIV status, examiner verified signs or recent use of psychotropics. In this cohort of men recruited as part of the Multicenter AIDS Cohort Study in the US, self-reported, rather than observer verified, physical symptoms appeared to be a primary factor associated with raised depression scores on standardised rating scales. The men taking part were approximately 5000 volunteers who were recruited from clinics and social organisations and through newspaper advertisements and by word-of-mouth in the gay community. According to the authors, they were representative of homosexual men who regard themselves as at relatively high risk of AIDS.

In cross-sectional work of this kind, it is difficult to establish whether men who are prone to depression become excessively aware of bodily function and appearance or whether such hypersensitivity leads to a reactive depressed mood. Social support may also play an associated role. Ostrow et al. (1989) demonstrated that social support played an important predictive role in psychological distress, and may have interacted with this form of self-absorption which leads to worry about minor symptoms. The role of social support will be discussed in greater detail later in this chapter. Contrary to popular conception, most people with HIV infection do not ruminate continuously about their health and thus, although the design of cross-sectional studies prevents the establishment of direct cause and effect, it would appear that over-concern with health in HIV infection is an important indicator of possible emotional distress.

In an interview study of gay or bisexual men under treatment in a university clinic in Canada, Chuang et al. (1989) compared 24 men with asymptomatic infection, 22 with AIDS-related symptoms and 19 with AIDS. It was unclear how subjects were selected, which casts doubt on the conclusions. Nevertheless, it was reported that high levels of psychological distress characterised all three groups, although this did not have a marked effect on functioning. As in the UK (King, 1989*a*), it was suggested that the extensive health care system in Canada, which is also free at the point of delivery, may have buffered patients against the effects of this distress. Interestingly, patients without symptoms, and those with symptoms of early HIV disease, reported higher levels of distress than those with AIDS, perhaps reflecting, as has been widely reported elsewhere, the experience of uncertainty and lack of resolution that accompanies the earlier stages of infection. Despite the infrequency of suicidal thoughts reported, one patient successfully took his own life eight months after participating in the study. Chuang went on to publish results of a further controlled, cross-sectional study, involving 47 well seropositives, 57 with either signs or symptoms of HIV disease, 40 with AIDS and 29 seronegatives considered to be at high risk through homosexual contacts (Chuang et al., 1992). Again, high rates of DSMIIIR Axis 1 diagnoses were reported in HIV-infected patients. However, most diagnoses related to alcohol and substance abuse, only ten subjects had a major depression with no difference on this diagnosis between HIV-infected and comparison groups. Furthermore, this study suffered from a failure to use standardised interviews and rating scales in the assessments.

Williams et al. (1991) have published initial assessments of a cohort of 124 HIV seropositive and 84 seronegative homosexual men who have agreed to participate in a five-year prospective study of factors that might affect progression of HIV infection. The study is limited by a reliance on volunteers recruited from homosexual organisations and newspapers, most of whom were well educated, successful and middle class, and by not including any other comparison group. At first assessment, the men had relatively low rates of current psychological disorder, most commonly depression and substance abuse. Although this finding is at variance with that of Atkinson et al. (1988), it may simply be due to what was considered 'current' in each study. Williams et al. (1991) considered all disorders in the month prior to assessment, while Atkinson et al. took six months as the defined period considered to be current.

Until recently, little data have been available from developing countries on psychological factors in HIV infection. We have just completed a cross-sectional survey of 164 homosexual men in Sao Paulo, Brazil, enlisting 42 HIV seronegative homosexual men and 32 men with serious blood disorders as comparison groups (Caputi & King, 1992). Structured psychiatric and social assessments were made based on those in an earlier London study (King, 1989*a*). Cognitive function was also assessed. Forty-four per cent of HIV seropositive men scored as psychiatric cases on the Clinical Interview Schedule (Goldberg et al., 1970) compared to 38 per cent and 28 per cent, respectively, in each comparison group. The differences between the gay men and the men with blood disorders did not reach statistical significance, possibly because of the small numbers in the latter group. Nevertheless, clearly there was little difference in prevalence of psychiatric disorder between the two groups of gay men. Important predictors of psychiatric disorder in the HIV-positive men were a history of psychiatric disorder or emotional distress, a family history of psychiatric disorder, alcoholism or suicide attempt, more advanced HIV disease, experience of discrimination regarding HIV or homosexuality, material loss through HIV and having had a seropositive partner. Although rejection because of HIV infection was associated with psychiatric disorder, overall levels of discrimination were comparable with or even lower than those occurring in Western countries (King, 1989*b*).

Prevalence of psychiatric problems in homosexual men

Several studies have reported higher rates of past psychiatric disorder among homosexual men, with or without HIV infection. Despite the limitations of an early study (Atkinson et al., 1988), which has already been discussed, there is other, more substantial evidence that homosexual and bisexual men who consider themselves at risk for HIV infection are subject to higher rates of psychological disorder. In the study just referred to (Williams et al., 1991), regardless of serostatus, 42 per cent of men were assigned lifetime diagnoses of mental disorders not related to substance abuse. Although no heterosexual comparison group was used, the authors took account of other epidemiological data, using the same instruments, in their conclusions. Perry et al. (1990*c*), in a study of over 200 people seeking HIV testing, reported that lifetime rates of DSMIIIR Axis 1 diagnoses were approximately double analogous rates found in the Epidemiologic Catchment Area samples, a large multicentre epidemiological study of rates of psychiatric disorders carried out in the USA in the 1980s (Regier et al., 1984, Myers et al., 1984, Robins et al., 1984). Homosexual and bisexual men in the sample had especially high current and lifetime rates of mood disorders and lifetime rates of non-alcohol substance dependence. Thus, although all people seeking HIV testing appear to be subject to higher lifetime rates of psychological disorder, homosexual and bisexual men report the highest rates. Finally, there is evidence that suicide is more common in homosexual men than the general public (Hull et al., 1988). This issue will be returned to later in this chapter in a consideration of the threat of suicide in people with HIV infection.

Until AIDS, study of the psychological health of homosexual men and women was restricted to samples of people seeking psychological help, and thus there was a clear bias in the direction of impaired functioning. It is less clear why lifetime rates of mental disorder should be so high in more recent, less selected samples of homosexual men, many of which are biased towards the more middle-class, materially successful, sectors of the populations. It might be that vulnerable people, who have suffered previous problems, choose to enter studies of this type as a vicarious way of ensuring continuing support and interest. It is likely that people of either sex growing up as homosexual in Western societies, which explicitly approve a heterosexual way of life, suffer many social and psychological difficulties. Their dilemma has been further exacerbated by the arrival of AIDS. If these reports are verified, the case for a more liberal system in schools and universities, which is sensitive to the inherent difficulties confronting young homosexuals, will become more urgent.

Prospective study of psychiatric disorder – incidence and risk factors

Studies with a longitudinal design are the most satisfactory method for providing information on the incidence of mental health problems in people with HIV infection. Cohorts of subjects are followed up over varying periods of time, and new episodes of disorder are detected as they occur. There are now several cohort studies taking place in the USA and Europe in which psychological factors are considered. Although most aim to establish the incidence and progression of neuropsychological difficulties in HIV infection, many incorporate some form of broader, psychiatric assessment, not least so as to exclude this possibility as a confounding influence in the development of impaired cognitive functioning.

An example of one such cohort will be described. Between 1984 and 1985, 1018 mainly white, middle-class, well-educated, gay men living in Chicago were recruited into the Multicenter AIDS Cohort Study (Kaslow et al., 1987). All six assessments were completed by 436 men over three years to December 1987. A questionnaire was developed for the study which incorporated other well-validated rating scales as well as scales designed to be specific for AIDS. The aim was to make an assessment of overall psychological and social status. It was claimed that the considerable rate of attrition of subjects with time had little effect on the findings. While psychological measures showed little consistent change over the period analysed, subjects reported increasingly intrusive AIDS worries. Overall, levels of anxiety and depression were higher than those for the general population, but lower than those seen in psychiatric outpatients. 62.5 per cent of participants *ever* scored positively on questions of the Diagnostic Interview Schedule adapted for the study, the Hopkins Symptom Check

List rating for depression, or admitted to suicidal ideation. However, only 3.7 percent satisfied all three of these criteria on three or more visits. Further reports of the same cohort have shown that suicidal thoughts are common with up to 19 per cent of men reporting suicidal ideas on three or more visits (Joseph et al., 1990).

Thus, emotional distress in this cohort of people with HIV infection, who had yet to develop symptoms of AIDS, was common but fleeting, rarely persisting beyond one visit. Only a much smaller group reported sustained depression. Subjects appeared to differentiate this dysphoria from more specific worries about AIDS which tended to persist and even increase in frequency with time. Unfortunately, no particular sociodemographic or serostatus variable was predictive of change in psychological functioning, although younger men exhibited greater general and AIDS-specific distress.

A recent study which depended upon case note data is of interest because data, which were collected in a controlled fashion on a very large number of subjects, showed a markedly elevated incidence of psychological difficulties in men with HIV infection. Prier, McNeil and Burge (1991) compared 573 American soldiers testing positive during the HIV testing programme in the US Armed Services from 1985 to 1987, with 2266 seronegative soldiers closely matched on several demographic and service variables. Over half the HIV positive soldiers were black, and 95 per cent were male. Ninety (16 per cent) HIV-positive personnel received at least one psychiatric diagnosis over the 30 months of the study compared to 36 (1.6 per cent) of those uninfected. Soldiers with HIV infection were five times more likely than their HIV negative counterparts to be admitted to hospital for psychiatric reasons and ten times more likely to be given at least one psychiatric diagnosis. Diagnostic differences, however, between the two groups were only significant for anxiety and adjustment disorders, and even this difference disappeared when those soldiers with CDC stage III HIV disease were removed from the analysis.

Thus, despite a greatly elevated incidence of psychological problems occurring in HIV-infected men, there was nothing diagnostically specific about the nature of those problems. While this report allows a direct comparison with an uninfected group of men, it is limited by its dependence on case history data and its location. Soldiers whose HIV infection is detected during Army screening procedures may be subject to greater prejudice and threat to their vocation than civilians who test antibody positive. Evidence for this is found in the authors' comment that, of the 17 men with adjustment disorders, 13 were hospitalised, at least in part out of a concern that a hostile or uncertain barracks environment might intensify suicidal ideas in HIV infected men. Unfortunately, no attempt was made to link the emergence of psychiatric symptoms with past psychiatric problems or with particular stressors which may have provoked the disorders.

Psychological health of long-term survivors

A group which are becoming of increasing interest in recent years are those people with AIDS who live beyond the normal life expectancy after the disease is diagnosed, normally about three years. There have been at least two studies of the psychological health of long-term survivors with AIDS, both from the Gay Men's Health Crisis, New York (Remien et al., 1991, Katoff, Rabkin & Remien, 1991). In a group of 53 men diagnosed with AIDS for at least 3 years, long-term survivors were reported to be resilient and positive in outlook. Only three men had a current depressive disorder. Denial did not seem to be the explanation in that the men did not think they would 'beat' the disease. They remained optimistic with a strong interest in the quality of their lives. It may be that long-term survivors are a well-educated group, adept at using the health service and thus a comparison group would have been helpful in this research. Nevertheless, as it is estimated that up to 10 per cent of patients with AIDS in the US live at least twice as long as the median survival period, these results have important implications.

Psychotic disorders

Most case series contain patients in whom a psychotic disorder is considered to have arisen on the basis of HIV infection. Hallucinations and delusions can appear as part of the clinical presentation of dementia and will be considered in more detail in a later chapter. Although it is frequently difficult to differentiate between an organic and functional syndrome, it is clear that a major psychosis can develop in clear consciousness in people with HIV infection, occasionally even before the appearance of physical symptoms or signs of HIV disease. Syndromes of a schizophrenic or affective type may occur, although manic presentations may be most common. Buhrich, Cooper and Freed (1988) reported clinical and social details of three patients who developed psychotic disorders, in one of whom the symptoms appeared before he was aware that he was HIV seropositive.

Similarly, Halstead et al. (1988) reported on five male homosexual patients who developed psychoses characterised by prominent affective lability. Prodromal affective and behavioural symptoms were observed between two days and two months prior to the onset of the psychosis. No clear pattern of precipitants were noted in this small series and, considering the relative rarity of such syndromes, the authors speculated that any simple mechanism for the production of schizophrenic symptoms by a neurotropic retrovirus such as HIV was difficult to support. Although there have been many other small case reports reporting similar syndromes (Vogel-Scibilia, Mulsant & Keshavan, 1988), we lack the necessary prospective epidemiological and clinical evidence to clarify the incidence and prevalence of psychotic symptoms or syndromes in HIV infection, be they associated with organic mental impairment or not (Busch, 1989).

Only one study has attempted to place such syndromes in context of a known population denominator with access to the same service. Kieburtz et al. (1991) described manic syndromes in eight patients with AIDS, which they estimated represented a fourfold increase in risk over the normal population. All were considered by their primary care givers to be cognitively normal before psychiatric admission, but neuropsychological testing after florid symptoms had abated revealed cognitive abnormalities consistent with HIV-related impairment in all eight.

Is there such a thing as an 'HIV specific psychosis'? Early reports concluded that this was unlikely. Later series, however, demonstrate increasingly that affective, particularly manic, psychoses may predominate. In my clinical experience directing an AIDS liaison psychiatry service in London, all patients who have been referred to me with a psychosis have exhibited major manic symptoms. These syndromes are not altogether typical of functional manic syndromes, however, in that irritability, rather than euphoria, is prominent, and patients are often left with residual distractibility and poor judgement after treatment (Kieburtz et al., 1991). The latter may well reflect continued cognitive disturbance.

Harris et al. (1991) reviewed 31 new onset cases of psychosis in seropositive patients, either reported in the literature or selected from a series in a San Diego medical centre. Cases considered to be due to acute organic reactions or drugs were excluded from the analysis. Initial neurological evaluation, including computerised tomographic scan and examination of the CSF, were normal in a majority of patients. Psychotic symptoms improved with neuroleptic treatment although side-effects were frequently seen. In 12 patients psychosis was the presenting manifestation of

HIV infection or acquired immunodeficiency syndrome. About one-quarter of patients, especially those with an abnormal CT san and EEG at the time of presentation of the psychosis, tended to have a relatively rapid deterioration in cognitive and medical status. This report is limited by the nature of the series. Combining a case series with all those reported in the literature until the time of the study is likely to introduce many sources of bias. Nevertheless, it raises the possibility of a direct viral aetiology in at least a proportion of cases of acute psychosis in HIV infection.

The underlying pathology of psychotic disorders in HIV infection remains unresolved. A psychosis could, in theory, develop as an extreme reaction to knowledge of the diagnosis, although this is unlikely to be an important explanation as cases may present before, or long after, the HIV diagnosis is known. In any case, the evidence for reaction to stress as a sufficient *cause* for psychosis in other fields is at best equivocal. Psychotic disorders may develop coincidentally in patients with HIV infection. Again, this is unlikely to be sufficient explanation as most series have reported a lack of family history of similar disorders in a good proportion of patients and, as discussed, there is some evidence that manic syndromes predominate. A psychosis may be induced by substance use which is coincidental with HIV infection and this possibility must always be entertained, as substance use appears to be more common in HIV populations in Western countries, whether or not the mode of transmission has been via injected drug use. Finally, a psychosis may be induced after central nervous system invasion by HIV, in the absence of a clear dementing process. Most HIV patients who develop a psychosis also show signs consistent with an incipient dementing process, and thus involvement of HIV is a strong possibility (Vogel-Scibilia et al., 1988, Kieburtz et al., 1991). On current knowledge, it is probably safer to regard most florid psychoses which develop during the course of HIV disease as categories of organic hallucinatory, delusional and mood syndromes.

Personality disorder

Despite much anecdotal reporting by mental health workers that major personality problems may arise, little is written about personality disorder in people with HIV infection. One reason is the difficulty inherent to research and clinical observation in this area. Delineation of abnormal personality remains one of the most contentious areas of psychiatric nosology. Psychiatric classification systems for abnormal personality enshrined in the

DSMIIIR and ICD10 are subject to considerable theoretical dispute and diagnostic overlap (Ferguson & Tyrer, 1988). It takes extensive knowledge of a patient's attitudes, emotions and behaviour before a secure diagnosis of personality disorder is possible. Thus, most cross-sectional studies obtain insufficient information on which to base such a diagnosis. Although personality 'changes' are sometimes referred to in series of patients referred to psychiatry (Seth et al., 1991), very few clinical reports have mentioned personality disorders. One exception comes from a controlled study of psychiatric liaison referrals, referred to earlier in the chapter (Ellis et al., 1992). A diagnosis of personality disorder was made in 23 per cent of patients with HIV infection, but also in 15 per cent of referrals from other medical units, a non-significant difference.

If this figure of about one-fifth is confirmed in other studies, it represents a considerable work load for the mental health team. Patients with personality disorders who contract a serious and possibly terminal infection are likely to regress to even less predictable patterns of behaviour in the face of this added stress (Seth et al., 1991). My clinical impression is that such patients demand an enormous amount of time, often with an unsatisfactory outcome for both the AIDS team and psychiatry.

Mr Q. is a 22 year-old, gay seropositive man born in Northern England who has lived in London for 4 years. He has little memory of his father who was last known to be in prison. Although his birth and infancy appeared to be relatively normal, behavioural problems in the home and school setting arose in early childhood and persisted throughout his teens. He was moved through a series of special schools to control his behaviour, and was finally placed under the supervision of the local authority as his care was considered out of control. He would often run away and hitch rides in order to find men for sex, but denies ever working as a rent boy. At one point, in an attempt to control his repeated absconding, he was briefly placed with severely abnormal adolescent offenders in a locked facility despite not having been charged with any offence. He received little effective education or other training and has never worked. Although he has little contact with his mother and stepfather because of his poor relationship with the latter, he remains emotionally close to his mother. He has had multiple homosexual partners since his early teens, never sustaining a relationship for more than a few months. He describes a chronic sense of boredom and emptiness and frequently binges on large quantities of alcohol. He has never abused other drugs. When referred to me, he had been made aware of his antibody status after a test consequent on minor physical symptoms some six months earlier. Since the HIV test, his mood had been labile with frequent outbursts of violence against property. He continued to have sex with multiple, often anonymous, partners but maintained that he always informed them of his serostatus. Although admitting to feelings of fear and anger, he was not clinically depressed and was given the DSMIIIR diagnoses of Borderline Personality Disorder and Alcohol Abuse. Although barely engaging with therapy, he consumes large amounts of time, and his sexual behaviour engenders anxiety in the medical team. The aim of management is to build up a therapeutic alliance that he may use as support at times of crisis, and to enable him to control his sexual behaviour. Low dose neuroleptic medication helps him to control his behaviour from time to time when it becomes extreme.

Why there should be a raised prevalence of personality disorder among patients with HIV infection remains uncertain. Substance abusing populations may be more likely to contain people with abnormal personalities, and people with erratic and impulsive behaviour may place themselves at greater than average risk in sexual encounters. Whether having a personality disorder makes one more likely to carry out risky behaviours is a crucial issue, but one which remains entirely speculative.

Suicide in people with HIV infection

Although it was considered that suicidal impulses were common in people who were aware of their positive serostatus, completed acts were thought to be uncommon except possibly among people with personality disorders in which self-destructive impulses were more evident (Holland & Tross, 1985, Faulstich, 1987). Furthermore, it was demonstrated that, at least in the short term, testing seropositive does not lead to a raised risk of suicide (see Chapter 2). Evidence accruing in the late 1980s, however, has demonstrated that there is a definite risk of suicide in patients with active HIV disease. Marzuk et al. (1988), in what has become a widely quoted study, reviewed all cases of suicide in New York City during 1985 in an attempt to determine how many were AIDS related. Rates of suicide for people with AIDS were 66 times higher than in the general population of the City and men with AIDS aged 20 to 59 years were 36 times more likely to commit suicide than their counterparts without such a diagnosis. Half of the people in the sample had expressed suicidal intent and one-quarter killed themselves by jumping from the windows of medical units in general hospitals. Statistics based on death certification may underestimate the rate of deaths due either to suicide or AIDS (King, 1989*c*) and thus these figures are likely to be a lowest estimate of the true rate. There were, none the less, several other problems with this data. The method by which rates were estimated have been criticised (Beltangady, 1988). There is other evidence that suicide rates among homosexual men, who made up the majority of the AIDS deaths in Marzuk et al.'s study, are higher than among the general public, possibly confounding the findings (Hull et al., 1988). Finally, no attempt was made to estimate the psychological status of people prior to their suicide.

Evidence from Scandinavia also indicates that the suicide rate in people with HIV infection is increasing. A systematic investigation of medico-legal autopsy cases with regard to HIV infection was carried out in Stockholm for the period July 1, 1985 to June 30, 1990 (Rajs & Fugelstad, 1991). These concerned sudden deaths outside hospital as a result of violence or other cause where previous disease was unknown or where there were suspicious circumstances. The data covered 96 per cent of all suicides in a closely demarcated area of Sweden but were somewhat complicated in that samples for HIV antibody testing were taken consistently only in the final 33 months of the study. During the five years of the study, 21 people with HIV infection committed suicide, 12 of whom were homosexual and bisexual men, eight drug users and one who had acquired HIV via a blood transfusion. Suicides among drug users were, if anything, lower than figures for the same region ten years earlier, before AIDS. Suicide rates for homosexual and bisexual men, before the AIDS epidemic in Sweden, were not available. However, the number of suicides among HIV seropositive homosexual and bisexual men increased during the study period, while the number of new cases of AIDS in this population actually decreased. Thus the proportion of gay men with HIV infection who were taking their own lives may have been increasing. Homosexual men most likely to be included in the deaths by suicide were non-Swedes, in many cases with weak social networks and lacking social support. Four of the gay men had case histories indicating major mental illness before the infection, and five took their lives when the infection had reached an advanced stage. A further 5 per cent of the people in whom HIV antibodies were detected after death were considered to have died from self-destructive behaviour, including alcohol abuse.

Two other recent studies are divided on the risks of suicide in people with HIV infection. McKegney & O'Dowd (1992) reported that suicide was less likely in patients with AIDS than in those with earlier stages of HIV infection, and that the risk for AIDS patients was even lower than in those who were HIV negative or whose HIV status was unknown. Conversely, Gala et al. (1992), in a study of 213 asymptomatic men with HIV infection, 123 of whom were IV drug users, reported that vulnerable periods for acts of deliberate self-harm were within six months of HIV testing and with the development of AIDS. Risk of deliberate self-harm was elevated by a factor of 7.7 for men with a history of psychiatric disorder and by a factor of 5 for those who had deliberately harmed themselves in the past. Although this was a careful prospective study of up to 42 months' duration, 53 (25 per cent) men dropped out, most of whom were drug users. It is always difficult to know whether drop-outs from studies such as this one are more or less psychologically robust. In this case, the authors assumed the latter.

Whether suicide should ever be considered justified is a subject for ethical debate. In Holland, euthanasia or assisted suicide is regarded as warranted in illnesses in which there is considerable, unrelieved suffering with little or no prospect of recovery. Although euthanasia conducted by a doctor remains illegal, physicians will not be prosecuted where it is considered that the patient has made a well-informed decision to seek euthanasia and repeatedly asks for it, there is no doubt about their wish, there is severe suffering with no prospect of recovery and all alternatives for care have been exhausted or refused by the patient. It is difficult to be certain of how many deaths occur each year by euthanasia in Holland. Although there have been estimates of 1900 deaths per year (Van der Maas et al., 1991), in a recent survey it was reported that 2000 deaths by euthanasia occur in family practice alone, each year (Van der Wal et al., 1992*a*,*b*). 'Pointless suffering' was the most common reason behind a request for euthanasia. In a study of 59 patients with AIDS, Van den Boom et al. (1991) reported that 60 per cent had considered euthanasia and 23 per cent had eventually undergone it. Main reasons were fear of dementia and physical deterioration. Although it was claimed that euthanasia did not adversely affect the grieving process of relatives, they found the sudden death traumatic, and there was increased stress where the euthanasia drug was administered by relatives rather than by a doctor.

Despite national views such as this, there remains considerable evidence that so-called rational suicide may mask a depressed mood, inappropriate guilt about being a burden to others, or an erroneous perception of the development of the illness and methods available to alleviate suffering (Glass, 1988). Although doctors in Holland must confer with a colleague before proceeding with a patient's request for euthanasia, there is no requirement for a psychiatric assessment of the patient, which could be regarded as a serious omission. Furthermore, there is evidence that Dutch doctors do not always comply with the requirement to consult with a colleague. In a survey of family practitioners, it was reported that 12 per cent of doctors had applied euthanasia or assisted suicide without having had any kind of consultation or discussion with a colleague, a nurse or with any other health professional. Forty-eight per cent had kept no written record of their last case of euthanasia or assisted suicide (Van der Wal et al., 1992*a*,*b*).

The American Medical Association (American Medical Association, 1992) has recently concluded that, although physician asssisted suicide may appear to constitute beneficent care, euthanasia cannot be condoned owing to the potential for grave harm. Instead, it is recommended that physicians do more to identify the concerns behind patients' requests, and make more concerted efforts to address their worries, short of assisting suicide. They add, however, that more aggressive 'comfort care' is justified, for example, effective analgesia which may have the side-effect of shortening the patient's life.

It may be that AIDS presents different problems related to stigma and dying in a young population. Studies of patients with other terminal illnesses demonstrate that suicidal wishes are uncommon (Conwell & Caine, 1991) and, although actual suicide rates are elevated, the relative risk is no more than twice that of matched populations (Allebeck & Bolund, 1991). However, many patients with other serious disorders are older and may be more certain of a supportive response from their loved ones. Debates about the merits or otherwise of rational suicide are taking place in many Western countries (American Medical Association, 1992), and carers for patients with AIDS may have to address the issue with their patients. Evidence about preferences for life-sustaining treatment of patients with AIDS, and those with other serious medical conditions can be helpful in this context. Frankl, Oye and Bellamy (1989) asked 200 hospitalised adults to complete a questionnaire on their views of life support treatment. Ninety per cent of patients wanted life support measures to be taken if their health could be restored to its former level, but only 30 per cent wanted it if they would be unable to care for themselves on discharge and 16 per cent if their chances for recovery were hopeless. Perhaps surprisingly, 6 per cent desired life support, even if they would remain in a vegetative state. A similar study was conducted with 118 male outpatients with AIDS (Steinbrook et al., 1986). Wishes for life-sustaining treatments appeared to be higher in this population with between 17 and 19 per cent of patients wanting major intensive care efforts even in the presence of serious impairment. It was clear, however, that many of the men were ambivalent about the subject, and often changed their minds. What was possibly more important than their specific views on treatment was their wish to talk about it. Seventy-three per cent wished to discuss it, but only one-third had done so. Most wanted this discussion to occur on an outpatient basis and thus, by implication, when they remained well and had had sufficient time to get to know their physician.

Such work illustrates that most patients in unselected populations with AIDS regard favourably those therapeutic efforts which are aimed at survival. Guidelines might assist carers in facing the issue. Most studies show that only a small percentage of patients who succeed in taking their lives have had no detectable psychiatric illness. Nevertheless, the presence or absence of psychiatric disorder is not synonymous with rationality. It is impossible to estimate how severe depression must become before rationality is impaired. Furthermore, when dealing with patients who question continuing to live, well-intentioned doctors and families might be influenced by their own moral views of life and death, or fears about aging and chronic illness (Conwell & Caine, 1991). There is a great need for public debate of these issues so that decisions can become explicit and take account of the views of patients, their families and their friends. This must be the case either for euthanasia or for the practice more common in many countries of withholding life-saving measures when it is considered that quality of life does not justify them.

In summary, perhaps the most important consideration for carers when faced with suicidal patients is to establish whether there is a treatable psychiatric disorder and, if not, whether the patient has a realistic idea of his or her future illness and quality of life. Mental health legislation to prevent suicide should be used sparingly, if at all. Considerable suffering may result for patients who are compelled to spend possibly their last days in hospital.

Social factors in the mental health of HIV infection

It is impossible to cover this enormous field adequately in a book primarily addressed at mental health. Many aspects of social factors which are important in research and clinical work in HIV are considered in their context in other chapters. Thus, only social factors of direct relevance to mental health will be addressed here. Correlates of mental health in HIV infection have received an enormous amount of study for a disappointingly meagre harvest of results. One major obstacle to progress has been the many methodological pitfalls intrinsic to research of this kind. Much of it takes place in a theoretical vacuum which has become isolated from the mainstream of social science theory building (Kaplan, 1989). In a detailed and thoughtful review, Kaplan (1989) highlights many difficulties which must be overcome. How do we translate theoretical frameworks of social causation into empirical questions, how generalisable are findings across cultures, what multivariate analytical strategies will permit an examination of direct and indirect effects in understanding the onset and course of physical and psychological symptoms in AIDS, and how can we introduce specific interventions and effectively monitor change and outcome?

The role of social factors, particularly life events, in mental health has a long history in modern psychiatry and psychology (Brown & Harris, 1978, Dohrenwend & Dohrenwend, 1981) Although research on the role of social support in the development and progression of disease had come under critical scrutiny in the 1980s (Wallston et al., 1983, Alloway & Bebbington, 1987), exactly similar themes were quickly taken up on a large scale in AIDS research. Support networks, coping, wellbeing and hardiness are terms readily encountered in the literature, but less readily defined. The difficulties in separating perceived from actual support take on less importance in the light of considerable evidence that it is the former which is crucial in responsiveness to stress (Henderson, Byrne & Duncan-Jones, 1981). Social support is generally conceived of along several dimensions (Zich & Temoshok, 1987). These dimensions are perceived availability of support, perceived desirability of support, frequency of use and perceived helpfulness, harmfulness or satisfaction with support. However, depending on a measure of perceived, in contrast to actual social support, even presuming the latter could be measured, introduces confounding influences such as current mental health and the independence, or otherwise, of events and attitudes of patients and those close to them. The result may be a collection of spurious correlations between variables which are not independent (Zich & Temoshok, 1987). Much of the work on social support postulates that support moderates the power of psychological and social adversity to precipitate episodes of distress or frank psychological illness. Evidence for social support as a buffer, however, is inconsistent, reflecting methodological differences between studies, but also suggesting that buffering effects are not of major proportions (Alloway & Bebbington, 1987). It remains unclear how much of the research on social support in AIDS successfully avoids these methodological difficulties.

With these reservations in mind, I shall take the risk of summarising. In many studies, perceived social support is correlated, not only with psychological wellbeing but, in some cases, also with physical symptoms and progression of disease (Zich & Temoshok, 1987, Ostrow et al., 1989).

Specific life events and chronic stress, such as bereavement or financial difficulty, have been particularly associated with physical and psychological deterioration (Baer, 1989, Rabkin et al., 1990). Contrasting results, however, have also been published. In a report on the Chicago cohort of the Multicenter AIDS Cohort Study, Kessler et al. (1991) concluded that there was no evidence that serious stressor events had any effect on progression of disease in asymptomatic men as indicated by a drop in T-helper (CD4) lymphocyte percentage. Life events were measured by assessment of numbers of lovers, friends and acquaintances who were diagnosed with, or who had died from AIDS over a six-month recall period, together with a checklist of other serious life events such as job loss or death of a parent. The authors went so far as to state that there was no need for asymptomatic seropositive people to avoid stress or to develop special skills for coping with stress in order to deter the progression of the infection. The issue of immunity and stress is returned to in Chapter 11.

A further difficulty in this work lies in its cultural and subcultural aspects (Kaplan, 1989). Patterns of social support are perceived and sanctioned in quite different ways in dissimilar cultures. Work in Africa or South America may have no particular relevance to Europe or North America and vice versa. The pattern of depletion of social networks observed in the physically ill or elderly, is unlikely to be the same as in patients with AIDS, or in those at risk of infection, even in first-world countries. For example, Hart et al. (1990) have observed that social networks of gay men in Britain are extensive, interactive and practical and thus, by extrapolation, are likely to be more supportive in times of crisis. In a study of 502 gay men, identified from community sources in several English cities, it was reported that the majority of men had extensive and supportive social networks. Although there are inevitable dangers in drawing conclusions from samples such as these, which are likely to be biased in the direction of individuals who are open about their sexuality and willing to take part in surveys, it was clear that the population was a well-adjusted group. One-quarter reported some involvement in the care of a person with AIDS, again reflecting the support side of their social network.

Many researchers have attempted to go further and construct explanatory models that are predictive of coping. By using so-called 'moderator' variables they hope to enlarge the proportion of variance explained by psychosocial factors. Unfortunately this work quickly becomes statisically complicated and difficult to apply to everyday situations faced by patients and their carers. In a study of asymptomatic, seropositive, gay men, Blaney et al. (1991) attempted to correlate psychological adjustment with stressful life events, social support and hardiness in a stress-moderator model. Hardiness is a concept that has been used for some time in personal and health psychology as a personality variable made up of commitment, challenge and control, qualities which are presumed to encourage cognitive appraisals more conducive to adjustment under stress. The concept has not gone unchallenged (Funk & Houston, 1987). Although finding that life events were associated with greater psychological distress, and social support with less distress, Blaney et al. (1991) could not confirm that a personality variable such as hardiness was a significant moderator.

One factor which is rarely taken into consideration in studies of social factors in HIV infection is the role of religion and religious communities. Little study has been made of religious or spiritual belief as it relates to wellbeing in people with HIV infection. One recent report at least describes the work of a religious community (Shelp, DuBose & Sunderland, 1990). The AIDS Interfaith Council of Houston is an association of clergy and laity which provides educational and service programmes related to AIDS. Although the programme was reported to be an efficient means of providing home-based care for people with AIDS, its effects have been monitored retrospectively, and no attempt at a controlled assessment has been made for the obvious logistic and ethical reasons involved. Difficulties encountered in the service related to training and support of volunteers, in particular there was a degree of resistance to the 'moral' issues of condom and drug use and to general aspects of sexuality. It is emphasised in the report that pastoral care and sacramental issues were available on request by the client, and that no spiritual or moral agenda was forwarded by any team member. Thus it is difficult to know what role religious belief played for either client or volunteer. Much more work is needed concerning the spiritual and existential issues that patients face, and how they might best be tapped in order to provide even more comprehensive support.

In summary, this complicated but fascinating research attempts to tease out the interactive effects of physical illness, past and current emotional disorders, personality variables such as hardiness and coping and social support. One difficulty lies in the divisions between research specialties. Much psychiatric research is carried out with scant regard for the complexities of confounding influences such as personality and social support. One current example is the World Health Organisation's cross-cultural study on the neuropsychiatric aspects of HIV infection now taking pace in at least six countries (Maj et al., 1991). Despite careful attention to measures of physical, cognitive and psychiatric function, little account is taken of the personal, social and cultural context in which the measurements are carried out.

Conclusions

Early reports of high rates of persisting psychiatric disorder in patients with HIV infection have not been consistently replicated in later research. Reasons for the change may have been biases of ascertainment inherent to those initial studies, or because discrimination and prejudice has eased in society as the infection becomes more familiar, and as public education continues to have an effect. In recent cross-sectional or prospective studies which have used standardised rating scales or interviews, prevalence of psychiatric disorder, variously defined, is in the order of 30 per cent or less. Although controlled comparisons are the ideal in such work, there are major difficulties in selecting appropriate comparison groups. The commonest diagnoses are adjustment disorders or substance abuse.

There is some evidence that lifetime rates of psychiatric disorder are higher in populations at risk for HIV infection, although these findings may relate to bias in the populations studied. In similar vein, although there is some evidence that personality disorders may be more common in patients with AIDS, comparison with patients with other medical conditions referred to psychiatrists do not bear this out. Nevertheless, such patients may present major management difficulties for mental health teams. Much less is known about the rates, or nature, of psychiatric disorder in third-world countries, although recent work in Brazil indicates that rates are at least as high or higher than in the west. Patients in poorer countries, who have less than adequate medical and psychiatric facilities, are likely to experience more psychological and social difficulties related to their disease.

Suicide is a definite possibility in HIV infection, particularly where there are advanced symptoms of disease, but at this stage it is difficult to estimate prevalence. Psychotic syndromes occasionally occur in HIV infection and may very rarely present before any other manifestation of the disease. Such syndromes appear to be predominantly of an affective type and are often accompanied by cognitive changes which may not improve after the psychosis has resolved. They are likely to be based on an HIV encephalopathy. Social support may protect people with HIV infection from psychological disorder but the evidence is conflicting and difficult to interpret.

It is clear that patients' social networks and degree of support will be important in determining their psychological wellbeing and possibly their physical status as well. However, study of these factors meets similar obstacles to that in other areas of psychiatry, namely difficulties of definition, measurement and assessment of outcome. Although the role of social support is yet to be clearly delineated in the AIDS field, it is clear that gay men appear to have wide support networks which are important in sustaining them if physical illness supervenes. Social factors are important in the emotional state of people with HIV infection and are considered in many contexts throughout this and other chapters.

CHAPTER FOUR

PERSISTING PSYCHOLOGICAL DISORDER

ASSESSMENT, DIAGNOSIS AND MANAGEMENT

Management of phychological disorder in persons with HIV infection demands a careful diagnosis. Medical and psychological problems may be complex and overlapping. The withdrawal and apathy of cognitive impairment may be misconstrued as a depressed mood. Management strategies, such as counselling and psychotherapeutic support or use of psychotropic drugs, are common to strategies utilised for patients with other major medical problems. Occasionally, use of mental health legislation may be necessary to manage deluded, resistive patients, but this occurs most commonly in the context of florid disturbance. Although the overall approach to the assessment and management of psychological disorders in HIV infection will be addressed in this chapter, many details relating to specific issues such as morbid anxiety about HIV infection, personality disorders, abuse of drugs or the development of severe cognitive impairment, are also considered in other chapters.

Referral to the mental health team may occur when the patient is depressed, behaves in a bizarre manner, threatens others or carries out risky or unacceptable behaviour which may be of a self-destructive nature. Referring physicians, nurses or counsellors may seek reassurance that their current treatment plan is appropriate or that the patient is not a danger to him or herself or others. The diagnosis may be presumed by the referrer who requests management with psychotropic drugs or specialised psychological treatment. It is unwise to accept the given diagnosis in such a referral and, as in all good mental health practice, a thorough assessment is mandatory.

Assessment and diagnosis

There may be considerable uncertainty about the underlying pathology responsible for the mental state, and careful differentiation of organic factors is crucial. For example, in patients who appear to be psychotic, a careful assessment of the level of consciousness and, although dependent on the co-operation of the patient, a cognitive appraisal should be conducted as early as possible. While patients usually undergo extensive investigation when they are known to be seropositive, greater difficulty occurs when psychiatric presentation is the first sign of HIV disease. Mental health professionals who may be asked to care for patients with HIV infection must keep abreast of the common presentations of psychiatric illness in HIV disease as well as with developments in the field of AIDS in general. Patients with HIV infection are usually knowledgeable about their condition, and expect carers involved in their management to be at least as well informed. As discussed in the preceding chapter, the most common diagnoses in patients referred to the mental health care team are mood and adjustment disorders. Psychotic disorders are rare and usually occur in the context of more advanced, symptomatic disease.

A careful history taken from the patient and from other informants, where possible, will also help to identify important risk factors in the past and family history, recent stressful life events, the extent of perceived social support, coping styles used in previous crises, and the possibilities for placement once the patient is again able to live independently. The family doctor is pivotal in this context. So often the general practitioner is ignored when patients are admitted or seen as outpatients and yet paradoxically he or she can provide the mental health care team with a considerable amount of information on patients' past and current circumstances, methods of coping and attitudes to illness. Clearly, however, there is a need to establish that informed consent has been gained from patients before approaching other informants such as these.

Careful attention to current drug and alcohol use is necessary as many patients may continue to abuse substances while in hospital, occasionally precipitating psychiatric problems which seem inexplicable in the absence of information on their current drug use. This may entail taking regular urine screens for drugs as an inpatient or outpatient. Alcohol abuse is a common problem in patients with HIV infection and may lead to even greater immunosuppression in its own right (Dunne, 1989).

Performing a brief cognitive appraisal on *all* new HIV referrals to psychiatry provides a useful baseline for treatment and assessment of outcome. Although testing on a one-off occasion may not help the clinician differentiate organic from psychiatric disorder, serial testing together with monitoring of the mental state will often reveal the underlying process. For a fuller discussion of cognitive testing, see Chapter 5. The most useful cognitive tests for the clinician are those concerned with premorbid IQ, mental flexibility and speed of information processing and verbal or visual memory. The National Adult Reading Test (Nelson & Willison, 1991) correlates highly with intelligence quotient (IQ), and is said to remain stable in people with psychiatric or organic illness. Trail making tests A and B (Reitan & Wolfson, 1985) are a measure of rapid visual scanning and sequencing. Thirdly, a useful test of verbal span, recall and recognition memory is the Rey Auditory Verbal Learning Test (Rey, 1964). These tests are suggested as a short battery for the clinician which usefully covers a range of cognitive function. They are simple to administer and score. However, there are many other similar tests which are well validated and may be applied according to the preference of the professional. When patients are grossly impaired, it may not be possible to use these measures and simple tests of short-term memory and orientation, such as the Mini Mental Test (Folstein, Folstein & McHugh, 1975), may be more applicable. As the tests take up time in a busy referral schedule, it may take considerable self-discipline on the part of the assessing doctor to make use of such tests on every occasion. None the less, baseline assessments may be crucial in deciding on the nature of future events should the patient's mental state change or deteriorate.

Counselling

Counselling for patients with HIV infection is carried out by trained personnel working within the AIDS team (Miller & Green, 1985), and it is appropriate that the majority of patients receiving such treatment are not seen by the psychiatric team. Much has been written about counselling in the AIDS field (Miller & Green, 1985, Carballo & Miller, 1989). It incorporates both preventive and supportive elements. Further transmission of HIV may be avoided if those with the infection are given information and emotional support. It is only in recent years that counselling has come to be regarded as a discrete skill. Counsellors have emerged as a profession in their own right, with their own associations, codes of ethics and methods of working

(Gray, 1988). However, we are left with the largely unanswered question of efficacy of counselling. While the role of counsellors in medical settings has gradually been expanded to include the treatment of a wide range of neurotic disorders, unfortunately there has been little assessment of their efficacy.

Counselling means different things to different people and has been described as a 'trendy panacea' for a variety of problems (Rowland, 1989). The British Association for Counselling (1979), in its statement '*The task of counselling is to give the client an opportunity to explore, discover and clarify ways of living more resourcefully and towards greater well being*', makes no direct reference to suffering or illness in the 'client'. Borrowing from several schools of psychotherapy based on psychoanalytical, behavioural or cognitive models, many counsellors in non-medical settings appear to adopt a neutral stance of 'supportive listening' and, while avoiding giving advice, offer insight and understanding to enable clients to help themselves (Rowland & Irving, 1984). This non-directive form of therapy may be rather different, however, from that applied in medical settings such as AIDS, where many regard counselling as including education, problem-solving, adaptation to difficulties and direct assistance with decision-making (Miller & Bor, 1988, Seeley et al., 1991). Perhaps the single most important function of counselling as it is applied in the AIDS field is to provide the person (and, if required, his or her partner and family) with the time, in a confidential setting, to come to terms with the knowledge of his or her state of health and need for behaviour change (Seeley et al., 1991).

Measurement of the efficacy of counselling raises similar issues to those encountered in the evaluation of more traditional psychotherapies (Wilkinson, 1984). The usual objection to controlled evaluation of formal psychotherapy has been that classical psychoanalysis is largely directed towards complex intrapsychic events whose measurement poses major theoretical and practical problems. A study of counselling may avoid the question of intrapsychic events occurring during the helping process. Supportive listening, non-directive help or health education are simpler to define in terms extrinsic to the patient. The evaluation of any form of talking therapy, however, contains difficulties which relate to the patient, the therapy and outcome. Should patient groups be narrowly defined and how can they be enlisted? Subject recruitment into counselling trials can be difficult, particularly if inclusion criteria are narrow, or if patients are poorly motivated (Ashurst, 1981). How can we accurately and reliably define the content of the therapy and what measures of outcome are most appropriate?

Measurement of outcome for a heterogeneous group of conditions treated in a variety of ways presents many difficulties. What is the relative importance of things like behaviour change, insight and feelings of wellbeing? Perhaps of even greater importance are the ethical constraints in assessing the value of counselling. The process has become so entrenched into our HIV services that it has become impossible to mount any form of controlled trial to assess whether it actually makes a difference. Varieties and intensities of counselling techniques have been compared, however, in attempts to modify behaviour and to ameleriorate distress at the time of HIV antibody testing. They are considered in more detail in Chapters 2 and 6.

Counselling in Western countries takes place most commonly on a one-to-one basis, although work with couples and families is also important (Miller & Bor, 1988). However, this is not necessarily the most useful or appropriate form of intervention in developing countries. Unfortunately, few studies describing or evaluating counselling for HIV infection in developing countries have been published. A report of 74 patients counselled in a Zambian hospital in 1987 reported that almost all were enabled to share the diagnosis with a relative who then acted as a resource to mobilise help in the wider family (Chaava, 1990). In another report, 149 married couples with discordant HIV serology in Zaire were counselled soon after notification of their serostatus (Kamenga et al., 1991). Couples who appeared to be particularly vulnerable to emotional problems were further counselled in their own homes by trained nurses. Major changes occurred in the practice of safer sex and only three couples divorced. Although not a controlled evaluation, it appears that the counselling intervention may have reduced marriage breakdown and encouraged safer sexual behaviour. Seeley et al. (1991) have described a community-based HIV counselling service set up under the auspices of a Medical Research Council of UK survey in a rural area of Uganda. The counselling developed during the project consisted of information-giving about HIV infection and provision of support to those already infected. Counselling in rural Africa must take greater account of traditional family hierachies, the possible existence of beliefs in witchcraft and religious beliefs which focus on disease as a retribution for wrong-doing. Although many of the issues are similar to counselling in the West, usually families are much more likely to be involved. Sometimes, counsellors would carry out community debriefing sessions in villages where results of HIV testing had been given. Problems encountered in establishing this counselling service included responding to rivalries in the village hierachies which were disturbed by the appearance of HIV, traditional objections to counselling of families by counsellors who were considered too young, and a woman's intense fears of repercussions on revelation of her HIV status to her husband, even if it were her husband who had infected her in the first place (Seeley et al., 1991). This service was described in the context of a community survey of HIV prevalence, and thus cannot be regarded as typical of services established throughout Africa.

Psychotherapeutic treatments by mental health professionals

Psychiatric referral usually occurs for more serious psychiatric disorders or major behavioural disturbance when the diagnosis is unclear, or when more specialised interventions such as psychotropic drug therapies, cognitive – behavioural treatments or dynamic psychotherapy are indicated. Cognitive behavioural approaches are described in more detail in Chapter 2 in a consideration of obsessive fears about possible HIV infection. When patients with HIV infection are referred, there is little in the *form* of the disorder that differs from psychiatric problems in patients with other physical disorders (Ellis et al., 1992, Creed, Mayou & Hopkins, 1992). The *content* of problems brought to the mental health professional, however, may be very different. Issues of sexuality, sexual behaviour and drug taking are less likely to arise in the context of other medical conditions. HIV patients will often bring complicated issues to the therapeutic encounter such as unresolved conflicts about sexual identity or drug use, estrangement from families, friends or partners, fear of physical deterioration, disfigurement and death, and anger about lack of control over the virus and its effects. Mental health professionals must familiarise themselves with these crucial areas if they are to be of any practical help to patients. Anger and rage may alternate with periods of denial and patients may frequently drop out for varying periods of time. If there are associated personality difficulties, the best the psychiatrist may hope for is to provide low key support, intervening quickly and effectively if the patient becomes depressed or suicidal.

Alcohol abuse is a more familiar problem to the liaison psychiatrist and, although management approaches are little different in HIV infection, the imperative is greater because alcohol disinhibits the drinker, possibly leading to unsafe sexual encounters, and complicates his or her immuno-suppressive problems. Embarking on a programme of controlled drinking may be very difficult, however, for certain patients who after lifelong habits of heavy drinking lack the necessary motivation to abstain. Others, particularly those who see potential benefit in regulating their use of substances in the hope of boosting their immunity, may quickly cease drinking altogether.

Self-help groups in the community contribute greatly to the effective support of people with HIV infection. It is less clear, however, that group therapy for patients with psychiatric difficulties is always appropriate. For example, there may be problems introducing patients who are reluctant to disclose their diagnosis or other personal features of their history. They may be concerned about confidentiality and, although prepared to visit an outpatient department in which it is relatively easy to avoid interaction with other patients, are not ready to discuss personal details in a group setting. Particularly frightened or vulnerable patients may find confrontation with people with obvious signs of more advanced HIV disease difficult to deal with. Drug users may find group therapy reminiscent of the more confrontational, less supportive style more common in drug treatment programmes.

Providing psychological support for the terminally ill is a particular skill which may not be common to all mental health professionals. Although psychiatrists and other professionals should confront their own fears concerning physical deterioration and death before they attempt to deal with patients' fears, this may not be readily accomplished. Nor is it necessarily clear, even with personal therapy, how this can be achieved. Death is a part of human life which is never discernible in an absolute sense, and thus claims by professionals that they have come to terms with their own feelings about the issue may not always be based on good judgement. Perhaps the most important experience is to accompany patients through their later stages and to be available when they wish it. There is no other way to understand the fear and mystery which is so often present as patients become weaker and it is obvious that death is close. In my experience, the major problems which have plagued both the patient and the psychiatrist become less relevant and this is a vital time when listening is powerful and effective. For the uninitiated, perhaps the most prudent option is to collaborate with specialty oncology or hospice teams or hospital chaplains who have considerable experience of working with the dying.

Medical and nursing staff may also require considerable support in facing their dying patients, but all too often this is not available. Young patients form intense bonds with many of their carers which, when inevitably broken, extract a tremendous emotional and physical cost. What is known about this process and how best to deal with it is discussed in Chapter 10. Although there may be requests for the establishment of staff support groups, again the mental health professional should have a considerable depth of knowledge concerning group dynamics before too readily acceding to requests to act as facilitator.

Physical treatments

The use of antiretroviral drugs in the management of HIV encephalopathy is discussed fully in Chapter 5. Psychotropic drug treatment of organic brain syndromes, psychoses, major depression, or adjustment disorders in people with HIV infection is little different from the situation with analogous patients without infection (Sno, Storosum & Swinkels, 1989, Seth et al., 1991, Ellis et al., 1993). However, the spectrum and severity of side-effects may differ. Although drug-induced granulocytopenia is a rare complication of antidepressant therapy (Gravenor, Leclerc & Blake, 1986), little is known about its effect on the immune system. Despite many anecdotal reports of increased sensitivity to psychotropic drugs, particularly among patients with AIDS (Busch, 1989, Miller & Riccio, 1990, Seth et al., 1991), there has been little systematic study of these effects. One open trial of imipramine in 11 seropositive homosexual men who suffered major depression demonstrated that the drug was effective in eight of the nine men who completed a 12-week course (Rabkin et al., 1990). Although there was a brief decline of CD4 cell numbers during therapy, six months later cell counts were actually higher than expected. There was also no report of unusual somatic or CNS sensitivity to the drug. Hintz et al. (1990) conducted a record review of 90 male outpatients to two university-affiliated outpatient settings in the United States in order to study the type of depressive symptomatology associated with HIV infection and the nature of antidepressant treatment given. Forty-five HIV seropositive patients who were treated with antidepressants were compared with 45 patients who had no known risk factors for HIV infection as determined from their charts. Although depressive symptoms were generally similar in the two groups, HIV seropositive individuals reported greater decreases in sleep and appetite than those in the HIV seronegative comparison group. Imipramine and fluoxetine appeared to be the most effective antidepressants with the least side-effect ratings in both seropositive and seronegative patients. While this study was limited to a *post hoc* examination of the effects of antidepressants there was no evidence for an increase in side-effects in the seropositive men.

In a report of eight patients with manic syndromes and HIV infection, there were no reported toxic effects from the use of standard therapies such as lithium carbonate and antipsychotics (Kieburtz et al., 1991). However, increased sensitivity, including dystonic reactions which resolve only with withdrawal of treatment, has been reported with use of antipsychotics (Seth et al., 1991). My own clinical experience does not confirm this impression. In fact, I have encountered occasional psychotic syndromes, considered after full investigation to be occurring on the basis of an HIV encephalopathy, which have proved exceedingly difficult to control, requiring large doses of antipsychotic medication. Most people eventually recover from the acute psychosis unless more severe physical crises supervene. Cognitive impairment, however, frequently becomes apparent on clinical assessment or formal testing after the episode is over (Kieburtz et al., 1991).

There is little information on the use of electroconvulsive therapy (ECT) for treatment of major depression in patients with HIV infection or AIDS. In one report, three men and one woman who underwent ECT for severe depression responded successfully with no particular toxic effects. Although the authors made some attempt to assess cognitive state throughout treatment, unfortunately only the Mini Mental Status Examination (Folstein et al., 1975) was used. Although application of more detailed tests may have been limited by the mental state of the four patients involved, this observer-rated test of cognitive function is relatively insensitive to early cognitive changes in HIV disease. The use of ECT in demented patients is not justified and is likely to lead to increased confusion.

Prescription of benzodiazepine tranquillisers is a fraught issue. Although useful drugs for short-term sedation (King, 1992*b*), they should certainly be avoided in patients with a history of substance abuse. There have been no reports of idiosyncratic reactions to this class of drugs but they are used surprisingly often in hospitalised patients. Ochitill et al. (1991) reported that psychoactive drugs were prescribed in 89 per cent of patients admitted to an AIDS unit in San Francisco. Benzodiazepines were most often prescribed either as anxiolytics or hypnotics. Antidepressants and antipsychotics were rarely used. The commonest reasons for psychotropic prescriptions were insomnia, emotional distress and nausea. The most frequently used anxiolytic and antipsychotic medications were given in moderate dosage, while the most frequently used antidepressant was prescribed in low dosage. This raises some concern as to the effective treatment of patients. It is important that staff are sensitive to the possibility that psychiatric conditions, such as major depression, may present as insomnia or disturbed mood in order to be certain that treatments more specific and appropriate than benzodiazepines are not overlooked. If there are no important side-effects with antidepressant treatment, the drug should be given in appropriate doses.

The liaison psychiatrist may occasionally be consulted about the management of pain in drug users. Members of medical teams become either anxious or annoyed when they suspect that drug users are importuning for relief of pain as a ruse to obtain narcotic drugs. These dilemmas may be very difficult to resolve. Pain is a complex interaction of perception and emotion which does not readily yield to reliable assessment. Consultation with pain and drug specialists may assist the team in coming to a consensus. Unless there is clear evidence against it, the most appropriate course of action is to take patients at their word and to prescribe adequate pain relief. Moral indignation or a global distrust of people who use illicit drugs should not distract medical staff from providing effective and necessary analgesia.

Patients with severe personality disorders may constitute up to 20 per cent of psychiatric liaison referrals (Ellis et al., 1993). Unfortunately, there has been little attention to their management in the scientific literature. Occasionally, such personality disturbances may worsen when there is superimposed cognitive disturbance. Such patients are unreliable in treatment and may become difficult and demanding when they do use the service. They may be disturbing or even threatening to staff and other patients if their demands are not met instantly. Unfortunately, many do not accept psychiatric referral or assistance, but, for those who do, it is crucial to offer a low key, long-term service. Frequent changes of junior medical staff may interfere with this process, and more experienced professionals who are in post over longer periods may be better equipped to deal with many of the presenting problems. On occasion, particularly when there is a degree of cognitive impairment, judicious use of low dose antipsychotic medication can be very helpful for patients in preventing outbursts of verbal or physical rage.

Social support

This essential area of patient management is usually the prerogative of social workers, occupational therapists or voluntary carers who may not always be in close liaison with core members of the mental health care team. Nevertheless, the importance of adequate accommodation and social support to patients' psychological health is an aspect of care that must be continually borne in mind. Arranging for befrienders and home care support is usually carried out in the larger cities by specialist community teams. Frequently, however, in smaller or rural areas, family doctors or district nurses provide the greater part of such care. As discussed elsewhere, isolation, a hostile personal or physical environment or inadequate coping styles may all contribute to impairment of physical and mental health. How to alleviate such problems, however, is not always obvious. Patients may insist on returning to inadequate or harmful living conditions or resist all attempts to increase their social support by use of companions or home keepers. Unless such hostility occurs in the context of severe psychiatric problems such as a declining cognitive or mood state, psychiatrists and social workers should resist entreaties to resort to use of mental health legislation when patients seem to be unco-operative.

Mr W. was a 48 year-old, intravenous drug user who, for many years, had lived either on the streets or in a series of derelict, unoccupied houses. He had lost all contact with his family and, although reluctant to discuss details of his medical history, his familiarity with psychiatric procedures led staff to believe that he had probably received treatment in the past. He would be brought in by ambulance when in a severely ill state with HIV disease but, after effective treatment and a normal diet, demanded to leave hospital. On mental state examination, he exhibited mild cognitive impairment, and although somewhat suspicious of his fellow drug users, there was no sign of a major mental illness. He had little social support and never received visitors while in hospital. He lived in squalid conditions in an unoccupied house with other drug users, from which he rarely ventured except for the occasional meal. Although formerly a heavy user of alcohol and a variety of other substances, his current use appeared to be low and sporadic. He proved resistant to all attempts to rehouse him in more sanitary and safe accommodation and insisted on discharge to his current squat. It was decided that there was little alternative but to accede to his wishes and attempt to cope with the damage each time he presented. He eventually died in hospital during one of his acute admissions.

Legal aspects of care

Just as in other areas of psychiatry, mental health legislation may be invoked when patients lack insight into the nature and significance of their emotions or behaviour and present a danger either to themselves or to others. The type of action taken, and under which circumstances, will vary with the social norms and mental health legislation of each country. Particular problems may arise when patients are threatening to staff and where there is uncertainty as to which legal agency should most appropriately handle the problem (Thompson et al., 1986, Pinching, 1986). Use of legal force to ensure that patients accept treatment for their physical condition is not warranted under the Mental Health Act of England and Wales (Gillon, 1985, Anon, 1985, Department of Health and Welsh Office, 1990) and would be a rare event in most Western countries. However, dilemmas may occur when patients become too demented to understand that medical intervention is indicated to relieve their suffering. Although there are few published guidelines in Britain concerning this situation, a psychiatrist would be completely within his or her rights to admit the patient compulsorily to a medical or psychiatric ward for the treatment of the *mental* condition. Fortunately, however, patients in this state do not usually make concerted efforts to avoid treatment, and routine medical measures can be taken.

Management of suicidal intent may be different to that in other patients because of attendant medical problems. If the patient suffers from a mental illness and is a danger to himself or others because of suicidal intent, it would be necessary and appropriate to admit him or her to hospital compulsorily under mental health legislation. However, placement of patients can be difficult. As already discussed, under the Mental Health Act of England and Wales, it is possible to admit a patient to a medical ward for treatment of a mental condition. Medical treatment would then also be available for problems associated with HIV infection. Where admission to a psychiatric facility is deemed more appropriate, close medical back-up may be necessary to deal with HIV problems. This aspect of care is considered in more detail below.

Psychiatrists may be called upon to assess testamentary capacity when a patient's wishes concerning their will or changes to their will are challenged. When asked to make a judgement of a patient's mental state in the final stages of illness or after death, questions of mental competence in the realm of personal and financial affairs must be regarded in the context of local legal statutes. The law applying to testamentary capacity varies from country to country and even from state to state within individual countries (Spar & Garb, 1992). In general, patients are competent to dispose of their possessions if there is no evidence for a major mental illness (including dementia) which impairs their orientation or understanding of what is involved. They should understand what a will is, have a sound notion of their assets, know to whom they could reasonably be expected to leave possessions and the respective claims of each. Although patients should not suffer from delusions or obsessions which distort their judgement in disposing of property, delusions do not in themselves invalidate a will. Finally, the psychiatrist should satisfy him or herself that the patient has not been subject to undue influence (Rentoul & Smith, 1973, Jacoby & Bergmann, 1991). Establishing undue influence may be very difficult and may lead to protracted court battles (Spar & Garb, 1992). Every patient should be given the opportunity to decide for themselves and judgements as to the suitability of their decisions must not be made narrowly. Eccentricity, or a will made against the wishes of those closest to the patient, are insufficient grounds on which to regard the patient as incompetent.

Psychiatrists who are called to make these judgements should first determine from informed sources the nature of the testator's assets and, if possible the persons most likely to be heirs (Spar & Garb, 1992). Assessment of the patient in a detailed interview is crucial and it may be helpful to have one or two disinterested witnesses in order to avert any future allegations that the testator's performance was coached. Information should also be sought where possible from informants such as partners, family and even friends. Careful records are essential as it is worth emphasising that the doctors may be called upon to back their assessments in court if a will is challenged (Fraser, 1987).

Management on inpatient psychiatric facilities

Special problems may arise when patients with HIV infection require management on psychiatric wards. Negative reactions on the part of staff may occur, patients' behaviour may place other patients or staff at risk, either through violence or sexual behaviour, and sophisticated medical input may have to take place in an environment unaccustomed to it.

These issues preoccupied many HIV mental health care workers and professionals in general psychiatry throughout the 1980s and detailed discussions arose as to the most appropriate ways in which they should be handled (Catalan et al., 1989). There was considerable discussion about when it was appropriate to conduct HIV tests in psychiatric patients and how issues of confidentiality should be addressed so that maximum protection for all staff and patients resulted. Guidelines issued by the Royal College of Psychiatrists in England and Wales followed conventional wisdom in recommending that all patients should receive equal treatment, regardless of HIV status; knowledge of HIV status should be restricted only to those who *needed* to know; testing without patients' consent should be restricted to very special circumstances wherein staff or patients needed protection from aggressive behaviour; patients should be regarded as if they were seropositive if there was any cause to believe that this might be the case; all staff should be aware of basic facts on HIV, particularly aspects of infection control and staff who were themselves infected had the same rights to care and confidentiality as anyone else (Catalan et al., 1989). Very similar guidelines for outpatient and inpatient psychiatric units were adopted by the American Psychiatric Association in 1987 and revised in 1991 (APA, 1992*a*,*b*).

It is uncertain how much impact this professional debate had on the actual practice of mental health services. Some of the British guidelines were vague or already applied in other contexts. Who needs to know about a patient's HIV antibody status is open to interpretation and is, in any case, largely an open secret on most psychiatric wards. Many of the issues relating to dangerousness of patients, sexual behaviour on psychiatric wards, and confidentiality were already very familiar to workers in mental health, and required little adaptation to incorporate special issues related to AIDS. Moreover, many of the medical issues were familiar in other guises to liaison psychiatrists. Perhaps the most complex issues concerned dissemination of information about AIDS to mental health nurses and doctors, and the establishment of effective ways to liaise with AIDS medical teams when HIV infected patients were on psychiatric wards. Most services in the UK have established local methods of working, but effective medical input to psychiatric units which are geographically separated from medical units presents the greatest difficulty. The answer to the question of when to carry out voluntary testing for HIV antibodies in psychiatric patients has also changed. In the 1980s, it was recommended that there should be some clear benefit to the patient either in terms of his or her physical or mental health and that, in any case, psychiatric treatments were symptomatic in nature. With accelerating changes in medical treatments, particularly those of a prophylactic nature, there is now a greater imperative to be aware of a patient's HIV status.

Conclusions

Assessment and management of patients with HIV infection is very similar to that of patients with other serious medical conditions. Professionals should be well aware of current developments in AIDS, however, if they hope to appear creditable and effective with their patients. The majority of people with HIV infection are counselled effectively by support teams of counsellors and social workers, and psychiatric evaluation is usually only requested for more serious or intractable disorders where specialised psychotherapeutic interventions or psychotropic prescribing are indicated. As in other circumstances a detailed history and mental state examination is critical, including careful attention to substance use and an appropriate appraisal of cognitive function.

Psychotherapeutic issues may centre on unresolved conflicts about sexual identity or drug use, estrangement from families, friends or partners, fear of physical deterioration, disfigurement and death, and anger about lack of control over the virus and its effects. To assist dying patients requires particular sensitivity and a need for objectivity. Use of psychotropic drugs follows routine lines, with the proviso that extra vigilance is necessary for the possible side-effects of antipsychotic or antidepressant medication. Such effects may have been exaggerated, however, and it is important that patients are not prescribed drugs ineffectively. Legal issues may involve application of mental health legislation to occasional patients who have lost insight owing to psychiatric illness, and who present a danger to themselves or others. Guidelines have been drawn up by various psychiatric institutions around the world which are applicable to local circumstances. An assessment of testamentary capacity may be requested from time to time and it is important that psychiatrists are conversant with the medico-legal issues involved. Special problems may arise when patients with HIV infection are placed in psychiatric facilities. As well as national guidelines, there is a need for sensible local policies and effective education of all mental health professionals involved in their care.

CHAPTER FIVE

NEUROPSYCHIATRIC ASPECTS OF AIDS INFECTION

Early in the AIDS pandemic in the United States, it was observed that neurological complications occurred in patients with AIDS, involving both the peripheral and central nervous systems (CNS). This simple statement belies the subsequent controversy that accompanied many of the neuropsychiatric findings in patients with AIDS or, more particularly, in those with asymptomatic HIV infection. Of principal concern to the mental health professional are the potential for impairment in well, seropositive people, the nature of the encephalitic process that leads to cognitive damage, the clinical significance of any such impairment, and the management of dementia.

Before cognitive testing became common in research or clinical work, there was increasing evidence, based mainly upon case reports, of mental slowing, delirium or frank psychosis in patients with HIV infection and AIDS. Viral RNA was detected in the brains of people with HIV dementia in 1985 (Shaw et al., 1985). HIV enters the brain shortly after transmission, probably carried within macrophages which cross the blood–brain barrier. Virus released from macrophages may cause a clinical or subclinical meningoencephalitis from which the patient recovers. With a later fall in immune competence, HIV begins to replicate in the brain (Perry, 1990).

In an early report on the neuropathology of AIDS, Snider et al. (1983) examined 50 patients with AIDS who had developed neurological complications. A definitive neuropathological diagnosis could be made in 16 patients. Four types of CNS involvement were described: infections, tumours, vascular complications and an undiagnosed group of lesions. A subacute encephalitis was noted in 18 patients, ten of whom had manifested cortical atrophy on cerebral computerised tomography. Symptoms in this group had included subtle cognitive changes, malaise, lethargy, apathy and withdrawal from social contacts. The syndrome was characterised in neuropathological terms by cerebral atrophy and diffuse changes in both white and grey matter. There was myelin pallor and occasional multinucleated giant cells.

Two papers, also from the United States, appeared soon after and proved to be very influential. In a report on 121 patients who had been followed to autopsy at two New York hospitals, 70 patients, of whom 46 had suffered progressive cognitive impairment, were described in detail (Navia et al., 1986*a,b*). The other 51 had been removed from the series because they had suffered macroscopic, focal neurological disease or a metabolic encephalopathy. A systematic comparison between the cognitively impaired and unimpaired groups was conducted. Impaired memory and concentration with psychomotor slowing was the commonest early presentation. Early motor deficits reported were ataxia, lower limb weakness, tremor and impaired fine coordination. Behavioural changes also occurred, usually apathy or withdrawal, but occasionally frank psychosis. Progressive cognitive impairment in the absence of impaired consciousness had occurred as the presenting or only clinical sign of overt AIDS in 25 per cent of cases. In the later stages severe dementia with mutism, paraplegia and incontinence was observed. Only 10 per cent of the brains were histologically normal. Although the pathological changes resembled those described earlier by Snider et al. (1983), severity of change was not always correlated with the severity of the cognitive disability. Nevertheless, this constellation of signs and symptoms led the authors to coin the term AIDS Dementia Complex (ADC) as a syndromal classification. They also went further to suggest that milder forms of cognitive impairment might easily be overlooked or attributed to physical or psychiatric illness.

Neuropsychological and neuropathological changes in AIDS

Considerable work followed these early reports. The term AIDS Dementia Complex was criticised on the basis that there is often little correlation between ADC symptoms and neuropathological findings and the possibility that the syndrome is to some extent reversible. The facts that a dementing process may occur without the full syndrome of AIDS, higher functions are not always affected and the so-called complex of cognitive, motor and behavioural impairment is not necessarily present, have thrown further doubt on the validity of the term.

There is little doubt that CNS function can be severely affected in HIV disease. For example, seizures may occur in up to 5 per cent of patients with HIV infection, without identifiable brain lesions (Wong, Suite & Labar, 1990). The difficulty lies in distinguishing direct effects of HIV from the effects of other pathogens, particularly viruses. Despite marked signs of disease there is often little virus material isolated from brain and spinal cord tissue. Further neuropathological study has led to the recognition of an extensive, multifocal inflammatory process, characterised by multinucleated giant cells (from which HIV can be isolated), macrophages, microglial cells and lymphocytes. Reactive astrocytosis is also usually present (Lantos et al., 1989). Endothelial cells of blood vessels in the CNS may be affected, but neurons themselves appear not to be directly infected. Thus it would appear that neurotoxic effects are secondary, possibly, to autoimmune processes, interaction of HIV with other pathogens or release of toxic substances from viral genes or from neighbouring affected cells (Perry, 1990). Understanding of the exact mechanisms underlying the development of neuronal loss and the associated cognitive decline remains obscure.

Until recently ADC was conceptualised principally as a 'sub-cortical' dementia, to signify that grey matter structures, particularly the basal ganglia, were predominantly affected. This concept arose mainly out of the distinctive pattern of abnormality on neuropsychological testing which will be discussed in more detail later. Recent pathological evidence, however, of involvement of the cortex (Lantos et al., 1989) and particularly of considerable neuronal loss in the frontal cortex, sometimes in the absence of significant clinical cognitive impairment (Everall, Luthert & Lantos, 1991), has cast doubt on this idea. In a small, controlled, neuropathological study, Everall et al. (1991) reported that there may be a loss of neuronal density in the frontal cortex of up to 38 per cent in patients with HIV infection. Applying evidence from other laboratory studies, they speculated that this loss may occur as a result of interaction of the viral envelope glycoprotein, gp120, with neurotransmitter receptors for peptide-T and vasoactive intestinal peptide, both of which may be protective for neurons exposed to the virus. Alternatively, gp120 may interfere with calcium metabolism in the neuron leading to cell death. A rise of intracellular, free calcium has been associated with neuronal death from a variety of causes (Dreyer et al., 1990).

It is difficult to estimate prevalence accurately from post-mortem studies such as these due to the complicated, and sometimes unknown, selection factors involved. Prospective clinical work, however, has established that about one-third of patients with AIDS will develop a frank dementing process (Grant & Atkinson, 1990). This is almost always in the context of major immunological decline and associated physical complications. The stages of the complex have been described, beginning with minimal impairment and progressing to a vegetative state (Price & Brew, 1988). A recent, detailed study has further delineated the cognitive deficits which are present on formal testing in AIDS patients who are not grossly demented (Perdices & Cooper, 1990). It would seem that the ability to carry out routine mental operations remains essentially intact and that global intellectual capacity is not compromised. There is impairment of recent and delayed memory and learning, and abnormalities of central processing and mental flexibility, characteristic of so-called subcortical dementias. Despite the findings described earlier of significant cortical neuronal loss, patients appear not to demonstrate impairment of language, praxic, gnostic or visuoperceptive functions.

In an interesting recent study, Morriss et al. (1992) compared 20 homosexual men with AIDS, 20 men with multiple sclerosis and 20 homosexual men seronegative for HIV infection. The two clinical groups were matched for disability and demographic features; all were walking outpatients. The seronegative men were included to provide normative cognitive data. Patients were assessed in detail using well-established psychiatric interviews and a short battery of cognitive tests. It was reported that AIDS patients demonstrated significantly more mental disorder than MS patients both at the time of assessment and since the diagnosis of either disorder. In addition, AIDS patients had suffered more psychiatric disorder before diagnosis than the MS patients. Nevertheless, MS patients had suffered more affective disorder, including elation, since diagnosis than the AIDS patients. No information is given on the lifetime risk for psychiatric disorder in the seronegative, homosexual group. AIDS patients reported more psychotic symptoms and symptoms of irritability whereas MS patients had greater difficulty with concentration. Unfortunately the small numbers (for example, only three AIDS patients reported psychotic symptoms) and the authors' somewhat confused interpretation of their results reduces the usefulness of the study. MS patients showed greater cognitive impairment than AIDS patients, which the authors regarded as 'typical of a subcortical presentation'. However, they admit that their tests were unable to discriminate between cortical and subcortical types of neuropsychological disturbance. In fact, AIDS patients showed little evidence of cognitive impairment, which may have reflected the relatively small number of tests used as well as the relative health of the patient group. Despite these somewhat equivocal results, the idea behind the study is an interesting one and bears repeating with larger numbers and more sophisticated neuropsychological tests. More might be learned about cognitive deterioration in AIDS by a comparison with patients with other neurological conditions than by further assessments which merely control for HIV status.

Cognitive impairment in HIV infection

One of the earliest controlled studies of neuropsychological functioning in HIV infection was that by Grant et al. (1987) using volunteers who were clinic attenders or part of a cohort study. Subjects underwent extensive psychological testing which covered a broad range of cognitive function, including IQ, attention and immediate recall, memory, learning tasks, psychomotor skill and parallel processing. In this assessment of 15 patients with AIDS, 13 patients with AIDS-related complex, 16 HIV-seropositive men and 11 HIV-seronegative men, it was reported that there was a gradation of neuropsychological deficit from 9 per cent (or one individual) in the seronegative group to 87 per cent in those with AIDS. There was no significant difference between seronegatives and controls. The level of disability in the seropositive group was alarmingly high at 44 per cent. Magnetic Resonance Image (MRI) scanning of subjects in the two categories in which there was active disease also confirmed that cerebral changes, mainly multiple areas of high signal density, ventricular enlargement and generalised atrophy, were frequently seen. Although the authors claimed to have controlled for alcohol and drug intake, their population were heavy users. No account was taken of psychiatric factors or the implication of the cognitive testing for patients. Neither was it clear how representative the men were of each of the groups.

The findings of this small study had a much greater impact than they warranted. They caused consternation in medical and political circles and were in part responsible for the screening of personnel in so-called sensitive sections of American society, such as the armed forces. It was suggested that progressive brain involvement occurred in HIV infection, beginning with subtle cognitive changes early in the infection and ending with gross dementia. Although other work confirmed the importance of the encephalitic process in patients with HIV *disease*, the extent of cognitive impairment in seropositive, well people remained in doubt and became a focus for an enormous amount of research. Men and women employed in highly skilled professions such as medicine or aviation, in whom even subtle deterioration in cognitive skills was considered potentially disastrous were regarded, theoretically at least, as a danger if found to be HIV antibody seropositive. The US Defense Department announced that seropositive military personnel would be removed from sensitive or stressful jobs (Harter, 1989). There were calls for mandatory testing for people whose duties involved high levels of manual dexterity or mental concentration.

Assessment, defining impairment and subjective complaints

The immediate difficulty which confronts neuropsychological assessment in this field is the nature of the assessment itself. Where global impairment of higher mental function occurs in terminal states or in dementia, it is not difficult to delineate the extent of the impairment using simple tests of cognitive function such as the Mini Mental Test (Folstein et al., 1975). When more subtle levels of disability are sought, however, such instruments are inadequate and much more sensitive and specific measures need to be employed. Most cognitive tests, however, were not developed specifically for this field but have been applied from other settings. Changes may be so minimal that patients may not meet diagnostic criteria for an organic disorder, for example in DSMIIIR (Perry, 1990). Tests must be sensitive and specific enough to detect slight impairment and avoid confusion with other psychiatric or personality impairment. The educational level of the patient needs to be taken into account as well as the possible confounding effects of psychiatric illness, anxiety about the testing, use of drugs and alcohol, sleep deprivation and previous CNS damage such as head injury. Even when a history of psychiatric illness or drug abuse is controlled for, there may be a failure to make a current assessment of mental state (Wilkie et al., 1991).

No agreed definition of cognitive impairment has yet been established. Studies have utilised a variety of patients, and volunteers have been selected according to a variety of criteria. A wide range of tests with differing cutoffs have been employed. In any random sample taken from a normal population, a small proportion of individuals will obtain abnormal scores by chance. Although many studies claim to be controlled, they are in fact only partially controlled in using HIV negative homosexual men (Joffe et al., 1986, Wilkie et al., 1991). Very few studies have included heterosexual men or men with other serious illnesses.

Self-reported complaints are not always clearly related to objective impairment on cognitive or neurological examination. In several studies, patients' cognitive complaints have not correlated closely with objective testing. Instead, they have correlated with psychiatric disorder or health worries (King, 1989*b*, Wilkins et al., 1991, Herns et al., 1989). In others, a definite correlation of self-reported with real deficits has been established (Stern et al., 1991). Nevertheless, the possibility of developing a dementia is well known to most people with HIV infection, and thus cognitive testing itself carries a threatening implication for them. Even if patients are carefully screened for psychiatric disorder, or if control subjects are carefully matched for the presence of psychiatric disorder, the connotation of testing will remain profoundly different for those subjects who are aware that they are seropositive.

Evidence from controlled studies

There have now been several studies of neuropsychological function in patients at varying stages of HIV disease and in well seropositives. In at least seven reports, where similar batteries of psychological tests were used, there was little indication of significant differences between well seropositive individuals and seronegative controls, cognitive decline appearing almost always in the presence of significant immunosuppression (Goethe et al., 1989, Janssen et al., 1989, McArthur et al., 1989, Clifford et al., 1990, Koralink et al., 1990, Franzblau et al., 1991, Gibbs et al., 1990). All seven controlled for, or excluded, psychiatric and drug abuse factors in their design and three included self-report measures of current anxiety and depression. Koralink et al. (1990) included MRI scanning and electrophysiological tests of brain function in their longitudinal study over six to nine months, reporting that, although no significant differences on neuropsychological testing could be found, electrophysiological abnormalities were far more common in HIV seropositives than in controls, and tended to progress over time. In summary, these results are consistent with the concept that asymptomatic HIV infection does not imply the presence of measurable or significant neurological or neurobehavioural impairment.

In a further series of studies, however, significant differences have been reported between seropositive people and seronegative controls, thus confirming the early findings by Grant et al. (1987). Three of them (Perry et al., 1989, Stern et al., 1991, Lunn et al., 1991) involved homosexual or bisexual men and screened for past and present psychiatric disorder or symptoms. In Lunn et al. (1991) all neurological and neuropsychological assessments were made blind to the serostatus of the subject. Wilkie et al. (1990) and Carne et al. (1989) carried out similar studies but without making an assessment of current mood. Naber et al. (1990), although controlling for past and present psychiatric disorder, included such a widely disparate group of men and women, homosexual and heterosexual, as well as prisoners who were frequently drug users, that meaningful analysis was doubtful. In general, the findings of these studies were similar. Subtle impairment, usually of memory and speed of cognitive processing, was present in seropositive people who otherwise had no symptoms of HIV disease. Psychiatric symptoms aggravated cognitive functioning, particularly in the seropositive subjects, but were considered insufficient explanation for the cognitive deficits.

How do we interpret these conflicting results? There is little doubt that there are early physiological changes in the CNS which are measurable by electroencephalography (EEG) or by analysis of cerebrospinal fluid. It is much less certain how important such changes are clinically. The subtle differences reported are often of little day-to-day relevance. In the study by Lunn et al. (1991), impairment was noted in 35 per cent of well seropositives, but also in 20 per cent of seronegative controls. Miller, Satz and Visscher (1991) also showed that although 13 per cent of asymptomatic HIV-1 seropositive men showed abnormal performance on a computerised test battery of cognitive functioning, this was also observed in 14 per cent of seronegative controls. Highly sensitive tests may have low specificity.

Significant HIV-related cognitive disturbance usually occurs within the context of immunosuppression. On balance, there is currently no clear evidence to justify screening of people in high cognitive demand professions.

Drug users

Cognitive testing in drug users presents particular problems in that this group are already known to suffer greater levels of neuropsychological dysfunction than non-drug using populations. At least three controlled studies have investigated cognitive function in drug users. In Scotland, Egan et al. (1990), using a fairly brief battery of psychological tests, reported no significant differences between seropositive and seronegative drug users. All subjects, functioned at lower levels than expected, presumably because of multiple levels of deprivation, poor nutrition and the use of drugs and alcohol. Those drug users who had lower premorbid IQs, or who had received less education, demonstrated greater impairment. In the second study in the US, drug users were followed prospectively for a mean of 7.4 months (McKegney et al., 1990). Seropositives were found to be significantly impaired compared to seronegatives on three subsets of a brief battery of cognitive tests. On follow-up of approximately 50 per cent of subjects, similar differences were noted on two of the same subsets but there was no sign of any deterioration. Conclusions remained uncertain, however, as the authors were unable to control effectively for level of use of drugs and alcohol, follow-up was short and the attrition rate, a problem hindering all drug user cohorts, was high. Finally, and also in the United States, Royal et al. (1991) made a detailed and controlled clinical, neurological, neuropsychological and electrophysiological examination of 108 seropositive and 51 seronegative IV drug users. Subjects were selected from a much larger cohort involved in an epidemiological study of drug users under way at Johns Hopkins School of Hygiene and Public Health in Baltimore. Only two of the 159 subjects, both men, also reported homosexual activity. Eighty per cent were in the asymptomatic stages of HIV infection. Ethanol consumption was common in both groups. Neuropsychological tests used were ones common to many of the studies already described above. Subjects in both groups scored significantly lower on the neuropsychological tests than established norms for a cohort of homosexual men but there was no association between HIV serostatus and performance on the tests.

Again, it would seem that there is little evidence for clinically significant differences on cognitive testing between seropositive and seronegative subjects, but it is clear that IV drug users are already impaired, presumably as a result of the effects of substance abuse, systemic infections, trauma such as head injury, and nutritional deficiencies on the neurological and immune systems.

Cognitive impairment in patients with haemophilia

The neuropsychological effects of HIV infection in patients with haemophilia have been examined in at least one controlled study. In Germany, Riedel et al. (1991) evaluated 181 HIV seropositive haemophiliacs, in all stages of infection, and 28 non-infected haemophiliac controls, utilising a battery of cognitive tests they had previously used in a presurgical assessment of patients with temporal lobe epilepsy. Tests included measures of attention, visuoperceptual speed, perceptual interference, vocabulary, verbal and visual memory and a mood inventory which had been designed and validated in Germany. Each patient also underwent an EEG examination. Although there was a trend for decline in performance on all tests, except non-verbal memory processing, with stage of HIV disease, differences from controls were only statistically significant for Walter Reed Stage 6 patients. There was no confounding effect of depression. Similarly, EEG changes tended to be more common in seropositive patients. Up to 25 per cent of stage 1 patients had abnormal EEGs. These results are very similar to the controlled studies in other patient groups which have been discussed above. A trend towards diffuse abnormalities were detectable in patients with early infection, but changes appeared to be of little clinical significance.

Progression of cognitive impairment

Although changes found are often subtle, it has been suggested (Stern et al., 1991) that they represent a syndrome which, although not sufficient to affect daily functioning in the early stages, may be predictive of later cognitive deterioration or of disease progression. Monitoring cognitive changes on a longitudinal basis provides the best method to test this hypothesis. Siditis et al. (1989), in a study of 132 patients with so-called equivocal AIDS dementia complex, reported that one quarter developed clinically significant dementia within nine months and a further quarter within about one year. This, of course, begs the vital question of what is equivocal or minimal impairment.

There have now been several controlled, prospective studies of neuropsychological impairment in seropositive subjects. Several of the studies already referred to entailed a prospective method. Most have found little major difference in progression of impairment when well seropositives and seronegatives are followed prospectively (McArthur et al., 1990, Fell et al., 1991, Koralink et al., 1990, Riccio et al., 1991, Franzblau et al., 1991). Furthermore, there seems to be no specific change in neurocognitive function as patients progress from symptomatic HIV infection to AIDS (Dunbar et al., 1992).

Little research has been conducted into neuropsychiatric complications in patients with AIDS living in developing countries. In an attempt to remedy this situation, the World Health Organisation is embarking on a major cross-cultural study of the neuropsychiatric aspects of HIV infection in at least six countries. The study will employ cognitive scales standardised in the West and adapted for local use. No results are currently to hand (Maj et al., 1991).

Recent terminology

In the light of these findings it is clear that the term ADC is unsatisfactory. The World Health Organisation has responded by proposing the term HIV-1 Associated Cognitive/motor Complex (HACC) to incorporate all grades of severity (WHO, 1990). Possibly a more useful division between mild and severe impairment has been proposed by the American Academy of Neurology in which HACC is partitioned into the more severe HIV-1 Associated Dementia Complex (HDC) and the milder presentation, HIV-1 Associated Minor Cognitive/motor Disorder (HMCD) (Report of a Working Group of the American Academy of Neurology AIDS Task Force, 1991). Differentiation between these two forms of HACC is based on degree of impediment in domestic, social and occupational functioning. Patients with HMCD should be able to cope with the majority of routine daily tasks, only demonstrating impairment when subject to unusual demands. There is little basis to the terminology in terms of differential response to treatment, nor does it, in itself, advance our understanding of the syndrome. Nevertheless, communication between clinicians may be facilitated, and patients involved in research more consistently described. Unfortunately the old term ADC is slow to disappear and remains common parlance, especially among clinicians.

Assessment and management of cognitive impairment

For patients in whom cognitive impairment is suspected, it is critical to differentiate an HIV encephalitic process from other CNS pathology, much of which is potentially treatable. Besides HIV encephalitis, the most common causes of CNS disease are infections with toxoplasmosis and viruses apart from HIV-1 or HIV-2 (particularly cytomegalovirus) and primary lymphomas. In common with all assessments in liaison psychiatry where a cognitive, psychotic or major mood disorder is suspected, it is essential to make a judgement of the patient's level of consciousness.

Incipient, acute, organic brain syndromes are frequently missed by busy nursing and medical staff who attribute bizarre behaviour to psychosis, or withdrawn apathy to depression. The clinician should familiarise him or herself with a brief battery of cognitive tests which can be applied quickly at the bedside. It is important to consider premorbid IQ, verbal or visual memory, mental flexibility and speed of information processing. Among an array of tests shown to be discriminating in the literature, which can usefully be applied in the clinical situation, are the National Adult Reading Test (Nelson & Willison, 1991) which correlates highly with intelligence quotient (IQ) and is said to remain stable in people with psychiatric or organic illness, Trail making tests A and B (Reitan & Wolfson, 1985) which are a measure of rapid visual scanning and sequencing and the Rey Auditory Verbal Learning Test (Rey, 1964) a test of verbal span, recall and recognition memory. When patients are particularly disturbed or unco-operative, it may not be possible to apply these more formal measures, and simple tests of tasks involving short term memory and orientation, such as those entailed in the Mini Mental Test (Folstein et al., 1975), are more appropriate.

MRI scanning is the most sensitive indicator of brain disease. It is not, however, particularly specific. Up to 75 per cent of MRI scans may have at least one abnormality in AIDS patients (Grant & Atkinson, 1990), but many anomalies, particularly white matter hyperintensities in seropositive, gay men, are as common in their seronegative counterparts (McArthur et al., 1990). EEG recording may show diffuse bilateral slowing of activity, and changes in the CSF are also likely to be non-specific unless infectious agents are identified. The distinction between the various CNS pathologies is crucial, however, in the clinical management of patients with HIV disease.

As already discussed in this chapter, it also important to differentiate cognitive decline due to a dementing process from that resulting from major psychiatric disorder. It is well established that cognitive impairment occurs in major depressive disorder and in some forms of schizophrenia. Such cognitive impairment may be reversible on treatment of the underlying disorder. Distinguishing organic cognitive impairment from that secondary to a major mood disorder may present considerable difficulty. It is essential to search for other evidence of depressed mood such as inappropriate guilt, self-reference, excessive self-blame, and suicidal ideas. Indicators such as reduced appetite, weight loss, fatigue and disturbed sleep are less helpful in the presence of active HIV symptomatology. In fact, recent evidence suggests that sleep disturbance occurs early in the course of HIV infection and is not accounted for by psychological disturbance. Vague, subjective complaints about sleep or daytime fatigue are present in most subjects evaluated in sleep studies (Norman, Studd & Johnson, 1990). Whether or not these disturbances reflect CNS involvement or immune modification remains speculative. A recent, controlled, questionnaire study has highlighted the importance of fatigue and sleep disturbance, especially in CDC stage IV disease, but has failed to enlighten us on the specific mechanisms involved (Darko et al., 1992). Although over half of stage IV patients complained of problematic fatigue, only 10 per cent of a comparison group of seronegatives did so. When stage of disease was controlled for, CD4 and white blood cell counts, total globulin, haematocrit, and lactate dehydrogenase were medical variables predictive of the level of fatigue and the level of disruption it caused. Nevertheless, these associations remain speculative and, in an astonishing lapse, the study omitted to measure levels of depression in the subjects taking part. Thus we have no idea whether psychological variables played a part in the genesis of this tiredness.

Irritability, although often a useful indicator of depressed mood in other contexts, can be a sign of incipient cognitive impairment and is less helpful as a marker of depression. Relatives and carers may provide useful information and may be able to confirm subtle changes in personality or behaviour for some time before the acute event. Assessment and treatment of depression is more fully covered in Chapter 4.

Evidence from both indirect observation and controlled studies indicates that the antiretroviral drug zidovudine can improve cognitive impairment. In a retrospective analysis of a consecutive series of patients with AIDS, assessed at an academic centre in Holland between 1982 and 1988, it was suggested that the incidence of ADC declined after the introduction of systematic treatment with zidovudine (Portegies et al., 1989). This decline was matched by a declining incidence of HIV 1 p24 antigen in the cerebrospinal fluid, the expression of which has been linked to the appearance of ADC. In at least one double blind, controlled trial involving 281 patients over a 16-week period, it was claimed that progression of cognitive impairment slowed or reversed and psychological distress decreased after treatment with zidovudine (Schmitt & Bigley, 1988)

There is much that can be done by way of explanation and education in order that patients understand the nature of the problem. It is particularly important to emphasise that the evidence for progressive loss of cognitive function is equivocal. Counselling about this issue should involve partners, carers and families of the patient. Judicious help for patients to organise their affairs and make a will may be invaluable. In more severe cases patients may be slowed, distracted, forgetful and disinhibited. Patients with HDC are usually unable to live independently and may make even inpatient care difficult and intensive. Because of attendant physical problems, it is sometimes impossible to manage such patients on psychiatric wards. At the same time, medical nursing staff may be reluctant to provide care for difficult and disruptive patients, and other patients may suffer continual disturbance. It is in this particular situation that specialist psychiatric nurses who have experience of AIDS can provide an enormously useful resource not only in educating and liaising with the medical nursing staff but also providing hands-on specialist nursing care on the medical ward in severe cases.

In Europe, mild cognitive impairment not due to reversible CNS or psychiatric disorder, is generally considered unresponsive to psychotropic drugs, the side-effects of which simply worsen the situation. In the United States, there has been a recent vogue for the use of stimulant drugs related to amphetamines. Reports indicate that stimulants may result in qualitative and quantitative improvement in higher cortical function, self-esteem and independent functioning (Fernandez & Levy, 1990). In patients where there is more gross disorganisation, perhaps with bizarre behaviour or frightening hallucinations and delusions, treatment with major tranquillisers is indicated. Patients will usually respond to moderate doses of the principal neuroleptics. Small doses, which can be so effective in the elderly, may be less helpful here. Although there have been case reports of severe dystonic reactions (see Chapter 4), including the neuromalignant syndrome (Breitbart & Knight, 1988), to antipsychotic drugs, there is as yet no unequivocal evidence to suggest that these occur more often than would be expected. Occasionally, use of benzodiazepines may be helpful in dampening extreme terrors encountered in terminal patients. Oncology and hospice teams are more experienced in the management of dying than most psychiatrists and it is therefore important to act in liaison with these specialists, if available.

Recommendations for management of dementia in other fields, such as the elderly, can be very helpful. These include retaining familiar settings for as long as possible, maintaining adequate lighting, adhering to predictable routines and avoiding sudden disturbance. Supporting patients' friends and families can be a demanding task and, although it is usually handled effectively by physicians, nurses and counsellors trained in HIV work, the psychiatrist may be called upon to assist in the more difficult or distressing cases. This is particularly so where there is a dispute about the patient's ability to make a legal will and testament (see Chapter 4).

It must be stressed that severe dementing syndromes in AIDS usually occur late in the course of the disease when patients are physically debilitated and in need of considerable nursing and medical input. The fear that psychiatric beds would be filled with young dementing patients has not materialised. Unfortunately, however, placement of patients may be very difficult. A recent study based in San Francisco, a city known for its extensive voluntary and statutory facilities, demonstrated that up to one-third of patients with HACC suffer placement problems as a consequence of their cognitive impairment (Boccellari & Dilley, 1992). Difficulty in placement was directly associated with the severity of the HACC as measured by a rating scale constructed for the study. More than one-quarter of the moderately to severely impaired were living at home with no help or were homeless and living on the streets. Those difficulties most highly correlated with placement problems were home safety problems, wandering, confusion and forgetfulness. Management problems were also linked to severity of HACC, although end-stage patients were less difficult to manage, possibly because of increasing physical debilitation. If unmet need on this scale exists in a city with such extensive health care services, similar or worse problems are likely to be occurring elsewhere.

Conclusions

HIV enters the CNS during the viraemia of the initial infection, possibly carried by macrophages. HACC is a daunting possibility for all patients with HIV infection but despite measurable brain changes in well, seropositive people, significant cognitive impairment is rare. Clinically important dementia will occur in at least one-third of people with AIDS but it is a late development usually in parallel with severe immune suppression. The term ADC does not adequately describe the central neurological and cognitive changes that occur and is insufficiently specific. Although newer terms such as HDC and HMCD are more specific, our understanding of the pathology or pathoplastic processes underlying the deterioration in CNS function remains rudimentary. Measures of cognitive function best applied in the clinical situation should include brief testing of current and premorbid IQ, verbal or visual memory, mental flexibility and speed of information processing. It is crucial to differentiate an HIV encephalopathy from disorders due to opportunistic infections such as toxoplasmosis or malignancies which may affect the CNS. Use of antipsychotic drugs may be indicated in HDC or occasionally in HMCD when there is excessive irritability or disruptive changes in personality. Although stimulant drugs have been utilised in North America, they are not widely prescribed in Europe. Institutional care is indicated for patients who are too impaired to live independently, and management issues are similar to those in the treatment of other populations with dementia such as the elderly.

CHAPTER SIX

SEXUAL BEHAVIOUR AND BEHAVIOUR CHANGE

In no other medical domain has responsibility for personal behaviour come under such scrutiny as in the field of HIV infection. From the outset, behavioural and social scientists have been as important as medical scientists in contributing to the understanding of transmission of HIV (Coxon & Carballo, 1989). Although the role of behavioural factors in the illicit use of drugs had been subjected to considerable study before the advent of AIDS, knowledge of the social and cultural aspects of sexual behaviour was rudimentary. HIV transmission occurs in many different behavioural and social contexts which can determine who in the population may be exposed and how they might respond. Cultural factors are very important in determining the types of sexual behaviour which take place. For example, sexually active, homosexual and bisexual men in Japan are much less likely than their counterparts in the United States or Europe to engage in anal sex, the behaviour placing them at highest risk for transmission of the virus (Isomura & Mizogami, 1992). Even among those Japanese gay men who participate in anal sex, frequency of condom use is high. Unfortunately, this interesting prospective study gives us little idea of the intervening cultural variables which may be important in determining sexual practices. Nevertheless, despite the low seroprevalence of HIV in Japan (mainly due to transmission by blood products), such data on condom use would indicate that education about safer sex is reaching gay men.

Prevention efforts target intensely private emotional and sexual spheres of life, and thus particular sensitivity is required in the investigation of behaviour and attempts to change it. Whatever the method of study used, there will be inherent problems of validity and reliability. Although HIV infection is potentially preventable by behaviour modification, there may be little incentive for those who are already exposed to alter lifelong habits. Sexual behaviour is not always governed by mutual or rational decision-making, is frequently unplanned, may involve unequal power or control between the participants, and may occur in states of altered consciousness induced by drugs.

This subject touches on a vast literature originating from different disciplines. In many studies, samples have been small and uncontrolled, and unvalidated questions have been asked. In this chapter, I shall concentrate on those aspects of sexual behaviour which are of relevance to the *psychiatric* aspects of AIDS. Factors affecting changes in sexual behaviour of drug users are described in Chapter 7 and will not be considered again here.

Behavioural change in homosexual and bisexual men

As sex between men was identified as the first important risk behaviour for the spread of HIV in western countries, it is not surprising that this group have been studied in greatest detail. Behavioural interventions have been evaluated and changes with time and education monitored. By the late 1980s, it had become clear that a rapid and significant change in behaviour had occurred in the gay population of the United States. For example, in 1982, between 40 and 60 per cent of homosexual men in San Francisco reported participating in unprotected anal intercourse. By 1983 this risk had declined to 30 per cent among non-monogamous men and to 59 per cent among monogamous men. By 1986, a 90 per cent reduction in these behaviours had occurred (Becker & Joseph, 1988). Summarising the results of several studies may exaggerate overall compliance with recommended changes in behaviour, nevertheless the decreases in risky behaviour are striking. Similar reports have been published for homosexual and bisexual men in European countries (Bradbeer, 1987, van Griensven et al., 1989, Evans et al., 1989).

Although it would seem self-evident that sexual behaviour is influenced by many interacting psychological and social factors and cannot be studied in isolation, surprisingly few studies have taken account of psychological or mental health variables affecting the types of sexual practices and the likelihood of behaviour change. At least some account has been taken of the extent of homosexual men's identification with gay issues. Joseph et al.

(1991) reported on the relationship between risky sexual behaviour and three main concepts important to a gay identity: sexual identity, gay social interaction, and identity development milestones. The predictive effect of each of these categories on risky sexual behaviour was analysed at six-month and 18-month intervals. The results suggested that successful integration into a gay social network played a role in reducing risky sexual behaviour among homosexual men.

In a controlled intervention with 104 gay men admitting to high risk behaviours in a small city in the United States, psychological rating scales were used to gauge whether significant behaviour change had any effect on emotional status (Kelly et al., 1989). Although the intervention appeared to successfully reduce risky behaviours, success in behaviour change led to no particular emotional effect. The same group later published a follow-up on 68 of the men at 16 months (Kelly, St. Lawrence & Brasfield, 1991). Resumption of high risk sexual activity was associated with younger age, earlier history of frequent, unprotected, receptive anal intercourse with multiple partners, greater numbers of past sexual partners and greater reinforcement for high risk practices. Thus, not surprisingly, resumption of risk behaviour was most closely related to the strength, frequency and reinforcement value of behaviour in the past. Psychological variables leading to an increased likelihood of risky sexual behaviour were intoxication preceding sex, lower scores on a depression scale, stronger belief that HIV infection is largely determined by external factors such as chance or luck, and openness about homosexuality. This study did not explore the importance of the emotional relationship with the partner. There is evidence that a return to unsafe sex frequently occurs within a relationship which is regarded as exclusive and long lasting. Further discussion of the factors ilnvolved in reversal to unsafe sexual practices is continued below.

In a study of New York gay men conducted between 1984 and 1986, Siegel et al. (1989) reported that drug use during sex, perceived adequacy of emotional support, numbers of years of homosexual experience and perceived difficulty changing behaviours were important predictors of continued unsafe sex. Self-esteem and alcohol use were also important. Very similar results have been reported more recently. As part of the Vancouver Lymphadenopathy AIDS study, an ongoing prospective study of 1000 homosexual men, Brian Willoughby et al. (1991) studied a group of seronegative men who reported continuing to engage in high risk sexual behaviour. A cohort of 139 seronegative men who completed an index visit between October 1989 and September 1990 and who reported sexual contact with casual partners during the previous 12-month period, took part. Thirty-one 'risk takers' who reported unprotected anal intercourse were compared with the remaining 108 subjects of whom 72 did not engage in anal intercourse with casual partners and 36 always used condoms when they did. The risk takers were younger, of lower socioeconomic status and were more likely to use nicotine, alcohol and nitrite inhalants. In Australia, Ross (1990) undertook a six-month longitudinal study of psychological variables predictive of condom use and safer sex in homosexually active men. Variables associated with increased condom use included personality, particularly a more assertive and forceful style, which may be an important factor enabling men to raise the issue of condom use with partners and promote condom use in sexual encounters. Lack of change to safer sex was associated with dysphoric mood state and psychological difficulties, suggesting that some people may need psychological support to assist them to make the change to safer sex. It would appear that younger, extroverted homosexual men who use psychotropic substances, and who regard events as related to external luck or chance, are at most risk. Personality variables and substance use are factors at least as important in successful changes in behaviour as emotional status.

As already alluded to, alcohol and drug use are common themes in reports on subjects who continue to practise unsafe sex (Linn et al., 1989, Penkower et al., 1991). Recent research on beliefs about how alcohol affects behaviour, moods and emotions suggests that these expectancies mediate not only decisions about drinking but also the effects of alcohol exhibited by those who have been drinking (Leigh, 1990). Thus people may use alcohol to act out sexual needs. Use of alcohol permits activity perhaps not acceptable under other conditions, rather than simply releasing inhibitions.

'Relapse' of behavioural changes in homosexual men

There is some indirect evidence that trends towards safer sexual behaviour in gay men have reversed in recent years, at least in certain European countries and particularly among younger men (Stall, Coates & Hoff, 1988, Hunt et al., 1991). There are many reasons why such a reversal might occur. The strength of sexual motives, awkwardness of using condoms, possible resistance to condoms by partners, negative connotations of using condoms and the coupling of protection and health to a process which is usually associated with trust and intimacy, all mitigate against firm adherence to safer sexual practices. Use of the term 'relapse' to describe this phenomenon, however, has been criticised on the grounds that comparisons should not be made between current older and younger gay men, but between young mens' current behaviour and that of young men years ago. Examined in this way, it seems that behaviour is undoubtedly safer (Pollack & Schiltz, 1991).

Ekstrand & Coates (1990) surveyed the behaviour of 686 gay men in San Francisco between 1984 and 1988, focusing on maintenance of behaviour change over time. There were marked reductions in insertive and receptive anal intercourse over this time and most men were able to maintain the changes for at least 12 months. Nevertheless, 12 per cent of men returned to practising anal sex at follow-up. Younger men who, at baseline, reported more sexual partners, and who were less likely to have a friend or lover with AIDS, were more likely to revert to unsafe behaviour. The authors speculated that social factors related to relapse were greater impulsivity, poorer social support for safer sex practices, discomfort obtaining or using condoms, and unsophisticated negotiating skills in sexual encounters. In a study involving the Chicago component of the Multicenter AIDS Cohort Study, Adib et al. (1991) identified variables predictive of return to unsafe behaviour over a one-year interval. Interpersonal and social variables were said to be more important than personal attributes or past behaviours. The lack of importance of sociodemographic factors and personality variables may have been related to the homogeneity of the cohort. Furthermore, the so-called interpersonal factors included low assertiveness in negotiating safer sex and lower limit setting skills, factors which arguably have as much to do with the personality of the subject as with each specific interpersonal encounter. Serostatus was not related to relapse or maintenance of safer sex. Relapse occurred more frequently in men who reported having only one regular partner.

More recent evidence indicates that behavioural changes are relatively well maintained. In a prospective, questionnaire survey of 262 homosexual men in Boston, Massachusetts, McCusker et al. (1992) reported that 96 per cent of men had already introduced behavioural changes in their sex lives at baseline assessment in 1989 and 70 per cent continued to maintain these changes up to 14 months later. While 18 per cent had moved into a higher risk category, 11 per cent had made even greater changes towards safer sex at follow-up. Predictors of a move towards riskier sex were inconsistent maintenance of behavioural change at first assessment and use of alcohol or drugs before or during sex.

Other evidence further indicates that a return to unsafe sexual behaviour most often occurs within stable relationships (Ross, 1990). Partners may agree to remain monogamous and assume that they can ignore the requirement to protect themselves during anal intercourse. Obviously, however, there is a fallacy in *assuming* fidelity in stable relationships; people should keep in mind the possibility of breaches in faithfulness in any monogamous relationship. Most clinicians working in the HIV field have encountered HIV infection in men who have had one, presumed faithful, partner in their lives only to discover that the partner's fidelity fell short of what they had supposed. The health education message to gay men has to be one of safer sex in all encounters.

It is important that behavioural researchers and health educators who are active in the field of prevention develop and evaluate interventions directed at boosting long-term changes in behaviour (Adib & Ostrow, 1991). Further psychological and social factors which maintain long-term changes need to be identified. One particular example is that of norms promoted by popular and respected members of communities. In a study in the gay community of a small city in Mississippi, North America, Kelly et al. (1991) trained people, identified as popular opinion leaders, to endorse behaviour change in their peers. Two similar cities were studied for the purposes of comparison. Forty-three opinion leaders were identified from gay bars as those most popular and interactive with others. After training in the clinical, social and behavioural aspects of HIV infection, they were taught how to initiate conversations and promote health messages by way of ordinary social contacts. Homosexual men in these communities were surveyed about their knowledge of AIDS, sexual behaviour and views of acceptable social norms before and after the interventions. It was claimed that risky sexual behaviours declined significantly in the intervention city with little or no change in the comparison cities. This is an example of the intelligent use of psychological skills by health promoters who were regarded as popular providers of leadership in their community. Harnessing the competence of leaders of this kind can occur in many contexts, and may serve to provide long term reminders to people that behaviour changes need to be sustained.

Behavioural change in heterosexual men and women

There is less direct evidence from heterosexual populations about behaviour change as it relates to psychological functioning. Although public health education and specific examinations of controlled interventions have been extensive (Hooykaas et al., 1991), few studies pay regular attention to mental health variables. The reader is recommended to Wight (1992) for a full review of the problems related to promoting change in sexual behaviour in young heterosexual adults. Issues of most relevance in sexual behaviour, and how it might be changed, are difficulties in talking about sex, gender role expectations brought to the encounter, confusion between the use of condoms as contraception or as protection from infection, problems in purchasing, carrying and using condoms, the effect of the stage of the relationship on the behaviour and the power differential between the sexes (Wight, 1992). For example, proposing the use of a condom, other than for the purposes of contraception, can imply in either partner promiscuity, bisexuality, intravenous drug use or previous sexual experience with HIV positive people. There are also powerful cultural forces which shape the form of sexual encounters. For example, there is a general aversion to talking about sex, especially during the first sexual encounter in a relationship. Such factors may prevail in the sexual decision-making process against fear of a sexually transmitted infection, no matter how serious.

As with homosexual behaviour before the AIDS pandemic, the range of expression of heterosexual behaviour in the general population remains largely unknown and proves difficult to examine (Johnson et al., 1989, Fife-Schaw & Breakwell, 1992). Apart from the usual difficulties encountered in large-scale epidemiological work, such as achieving an unbiased random sampling of a population, or avoiding a low response rate, studies founder because of semantic confusion in the questions, or because their explicit content engenders high refusal rates, because there is scepticism about the validity and reliability of the data, or because funding bodies (on occasions even governments) recoil at the prospect of supporting the work. It is even unclear how best to collect information. Although interviews may result in more detailed data, potentially embarrassing issues may be easier to respond to by the more anonymous pen and paper method (Fife-Schaw & Breakwell, 1992). Without large-scale surveys of the general population, it is very difficult to interpret the findings of smaller surveys on special groups. Information on numbers of sexually active individuals at various ages in the population, numbers of sexual partners and frequency of sexual encounters, condom use and same sex contact is essential if the behaviour of sub groups of the population is to be placed in context. Summarising the little data that is available concerning young people in the United Kingdom it appears that 50 per cent of adolescents of both sexes have experienced sexual intercourse by the age of 16 years, 20 per cent of 16 to 20 year-olds have had a total of four or more partners, between 15 and 55 per cent of both sexes aged 16 to

21 years report using a condom in their most recent sexual intercourse, 8 to 9 per cent of both sexes have experienced heterosexual anal intercourse, and between 0.5 and 5 per cent report same sex experiences (Fife-Schaw & Breakwell, 1992). There seems little doubt that figures reported for activities which are more difficult or embarrassing to report, such as same sex experiences or anal intercourse, are underestimates.

Unfortunately, even in small surveys, little account is taken of crucial psychological variables such as insecurity about sexual identity, the process of relationship development, each sex's perception of the other or (particularly male) assumptions about the inevitability of the sex drive. Issues such as lack of confidence, fear of ridicule and an inability to express need, or lack of it, which leads to maintaining ambiguity about one's sexual intentions as long as possible in sexual encounters, have received little consideration in efforts to educate or change behaviour (Wight, 1992). More specifically, psychiatric factors such as anxiety or depression, which are often considered in the field of sexual counselling, are also rarely considered in population studies of sexual behaviour. Even in intervention studies to change sexual behaviour, such factors are often omitted. Most research has concentrated on special groups such as couples in which one person is infected with HIV or has involved large-scale surveys on general populations following public health campaigns.

In one recent example where psychological variables were explicitly considered, 149 married couples with discordant HIV serology in Zaire (Kamenga et al., 1991), were counselled soon after notification of their serostatus. Subjects were recruited after extensive screening of employees working in two large companies. Couples were counselled monthly, supplied with condoms, and asked to keep a sexual activity diary. Those couples who seemed particularly vulnerable to emotional problems were counselled more intensively in their own homes by trained nurses. Whereas before notification only 5 per cent of couples had ever used barrier contraception, 18 months later 77 per cent of the couples reported using condoms in all sexual encounters. In only six couples was HIV transmitted to the initially uninfected partner. Only three couples divorced. Careful attention to psychological distress in this study may have reduced marriage break-up and clearly encouraged compliance with the advice on sexual behaviour. In a recent Californian study of 188 young, heterosexually active, university students, the role of anxiety about contracting disease and antipathy towards homosexuality was considered along with other cognitive and behavioural factors, in determining sexual behaviour (Cochran &

Peplau, 1991). For both sexes, higher levels of worry were a significant predictor of risk reduction behaviour. For women, more active sexual histories predicted higher levels of worry about contracting a sexually transmitted infection, while, for men, perceived personal vulnerability and antipathy towards homosexuality were important. Personal vulnerability, however, was taken to mean the estimated personal probability of ever contracting a sexually transmitted disease (STD), or being exposed to HIV, and is likely to be confounded by many other factors. Negative attitudes towards homosexuality as a predictor of worry implies that care should be exercised in including information on gay lifestyles in AIDS education programmes targeted at heterosexual men. It also implies that heterosexual men may need to be appropriately educated about HIV transmission to counteract animosity towards their homosexual counterparts.

Psychological and social factors associated with the acquisition of STDs were studied by Shafer & Boyer (1991) in 544 students attending four urban academic high schools in California. Their data were collected at the beginning of an intervention study, and measured parameters of knowledge, behaviour and attitudes towards STDs and HIV infection. Although questions were asked about alcohol and drug use, unfortunately no assessment was made of the student's current mental state. A higher level of knowledge about STD and AIDS was associated with lower anxiety about STD and AIDS, fewer negative attitudes towards people with AIDS, stronger perceptions of self-efficacy and stronger peer affiliation. Alcohol and drug use emerged as the best predictor of sexual risk behaviours while lower knowledge of STD and AIDS, and the perception that peers were not engaging in preventative behaviour were the best predictors of failing to use condoms. Negative attitudes towards people with AIDS were inversely related to STD and AIDS knowledge, social support and perceived self-efficacy. Finally, the strongest predictors of drug and alcohol use were perceptions that peers were not engaging in preventive behaviours together with strong peer affiliation. Thus, these data demonstrate clearly that knowledge and behaviour with regard to STDs are closely associated with particular psychological and social variables which will vary with the culture in which the young people live. At least in the United States, students who were well informed about AIDS and STDs also appear to have lowest anxiety about them and fewer negative attitudes and are most self confident. These factors are crucial in attempts to educate young people in prevention efforts against AIDS.

The most comprehensive study to date, which has explicitly considered the influence of mental health problems on risk behaviours of young adults, is one in which 602 inner city youths were interviewed three times between 1984 and 1990 in several large North American cities (Stiffman et al., 1992). The data reported arose from a substudy of a larger cohort who were taking part in an investigation of the delivery of health care and social services. Just prior to the third interview, the youths were divided on the basis of their self-reports into *high risk* to mean those who had engaged in prostitution, injectable drug use or homosexual activity or who had suffered an ulcerating sexually transmitted disease, *moderate risk* to mean those with more than six sexual partners over the year before interview, or who had suffered a non-ulcerative sexually transmitted disease, and lastly, youths who were considered at *low risk* for HIV infection. Samples were then selected in a stratified manner for this third interview. Psychiatric symptoms in adolescence were predictive of later risky behaviours including engaging in prostitution, use of prostitutes, intravenous drug use, choice of high risk sexual partners and reporting multiple sexual partners. Although correlations were moderate, the strongest predictors of later risky behaviour were adolescent alcohol and drug use and conduct disorder. The authors claimed that their findings were not explicable simply on the basis that adolescents engaging in risk behaviours when first seen might later also suffer mental health problems and be likely to continue their AIDS-related risk behaviours. Most of the risk behaviours were initiated after adolescence. Although no specific treatment was monitored as part of this prospective study, a reduction in psychological symptoms resulted in a reduction in AIDS-related risk behaviour, pointing to the potential for intervention. The problems with this study were that the youths were selected from among health clinic *attenders* in cities with high rates of homicide, suicide and drug use and thus were unlikely to be representative of all youths from such areas. Drop-out at each interview may also have been more likely in higher risk individuals. Finally, stratified sampling of higher risk individuals contains an inherent risk of exaggerating correlations in the total sample. Nevertheless, the study provides compelling evidence that mental health is a crucial predictor of AIDS-related risk behaviours in young people living in inner cities, and indicates that prevention efforts targeted at mental health are likely to have greater success in reducing risky behaviours than continued efforts to increase the knowledge base of an already reasonably well-informed population.

Studies of the effects of drugs and alcohol on sexual behaviour of heterosexual men and women show similar patterns to that in homosexuals.

In fact, for some years, it has been well known that alcohol and other psychotropic drugs are associated with disinhibited sexual behaviour (Soloman & Andrews, 1973). In a large study of young people in Scotland, interviewed while at school between 1979 and 1983, and followed up between 1988 and 1989, Bagnall, Plant and Warwick (1990) reported that, although actual levels of alcohol consumption were not associated with condom use or number of sexual partners, subjects who often combined alcohol and sex were seven times less likely than others to report always using condoms for vaginal intercourse. Other mental health problems may intervene on the pathway to high risk behaviours. It has been demonstrated in adolescents that depression is a potent predictor of alcohol and drug abuse (Deykin, Levy & Wells, 1987).

In a recent prospective study of the effect of counselling and educational interventions on transmission in couples discordant for HIV infection in Rwanda (Allen et al., 1992) it was reported that, in all of the discordant couples in which the HIV seronegative partner seroconverted during the time of the study, the man was reported to drink alcohol regularly. Clearly, education on safer sex practices is insufficient alone to prevent risky behaviour. Use of alcohol, particularly by the male partner, may disrupt attempts at safe sex even when each member of the couple is fully cognisant of the risk.

Finally, it must be reiterated that studies of sexual behaviour are only as good as the accuracy of the self-reports on which they are based. Studies of agreement between members of couples are conflicting in their conclusions. Padian (1990), in a study of 98 heterosexual couples in which each member was interviewed separately, reported that there was reasonably high agreement between them (Kappas greater than 0.7) on the number of vaginal intercourse contacts, condom use, and the practice of anal intercourse. However, the couples, who were volunteers, knew beforehand that they were to interviewed about their sex lives and may have had time for discussion. Enlisting a more marginalised group, Kleyn, Day and Weis (1991) reported on the sexual behaviour of 143 monogamous couples who took part in a study of treatment of intravenous drug users and their non-injecting partner. Intravenous drug users' self-reports of their sexual behaviour were compared with those of their sexual partners. When partners were interviewed separately, major discrepancies were found in agreement on frequency of use of birth control or condoms, vaginal sex, oral sex or anal sex. Although these results serve as a reminder of the inherent unreliability of reported sexual behaviour, there were problems with the study. The information was collected in 26 separate sites which left room for error. Furthermore, degree of concordance of reported sexual behaviour between members of a couple will depend on how frequently that behaviour occurs. For example, anal sex was rarely reported and therefore agreement on its occurrence and non-occurrence might be relatively high. Vaginal sex, in contrast, had a very low agreement (24.4 per cent) perhaps merely because it is a more common behaviour and less readily remembered by either one of the couple. Sexual behaviour is difficult to measure, let alone change.

Sex workers

People who have sex for money or other commercial gain, such as drugs, have long been a focus for preventive efforts against HIV infection. However, recruiting prostitutes into studies is difficult because of the stigmatised and sometimes illegal nature of their work. There has also been concern to avoid scapegoating prostitutes by exaggerating their role as sources of infection. From social and anthropological perspectives prostitution is an immensely complex phenomenon varying across the sexes and across cultures. Over the past 20 years, there has been a move to reduce the stigma of prostitution, by reconceptualising prostitutes as sex workers in a wider sex industry. The behaviour of sex workers varies enormously depending on whether they are male, female or transsexual, their place of work, the nature and demands of their clientele, any associated drug use and the legal constraints and cultural context within which they work and live (Day, 1988). Thus it is impossible to summarise the place of the sex worker in the AIDS pandemic.

Seroprevalence in female prostitutes varies widely between countries and studies. In sub-Saharan Africa, rates reported have varied between 1 and 88 per cent (Campbell, 1990). Although the findings are very difficult to interpret because of selection factors and the background seroprevalence of the country concerned, it would appear that, in this context, casual or professional prostitute women and their clients play an important role in the transmission of HIV infection. Just as importantly, it is clear that educational interventions can markedly increase frequency of protected sex in this group (Ngugi et al., 1988). In the West, prevalence of HIV infection among female sex workers is generally low, unless there is attendant drug use, and condom use is high. Screening of 114 intravenous drug using and 190 non-using female prostitutes in several Italian cities revealed HIV antibodies in 36 per cent of the former but in only 1.6 per cent of the latter (Tirelli et al., 1989). In a follow-up study of 91 female prostitutes over 17 months in a London STD clinic, 75 per cent of the women were using condoms with all clients by late 1987, whereas only 9 per cent were always using condoms with boyfriends. Seroprevalence of HIV for prostitutes in this same clinic stood at 1.6 per cent, all of whom had been involved in drug use or had had an HIV positive boyfriend (Day, Wrad & Harris, 1988). It is clear that prostitutes may be placing themselves at greatest risk from unprotected sex with boyfriends.

The question of whether sex workers actually confer an elevated risk of HIV infection on their clients depends on the context and culture in which the prostitution takes place. Reports of clients cannot be relied upon. A number of men who learn that they are seropositive may prefer to admit to contact with prostitutes than sex with other men, particularly in special situations where homosexual activity is proscribed (Potterat, Phillips & Muth, 1987). Similar accounts may be given by men who are embarrassed to admit to homosexual behaviour when receiving treatment from a clinic for sexually transmitted diseases.

Studies of the behaviour of prostitutes and other sex workers, such as escorts, have often failed to take account of mental health factors despite the obvious fact that many people in this industry are socially and economically deprived, are often heavily dependent on third parties to recruit clients and may have been subjected to major mental health stressors in childhood or as young adults. For example, in a study of approximately 3000 prostitutes in the United States, it was reported that months of i.v. drug use, presence of seromarkers for hepatitis infection, being a member of a minority ethnic group and infrequent use of condoms with *partners*, in contrast to customers, were significant independent predictors of HIV infection (Campbell, 1990). However, no account was taken of psychological and personality variables which may be crucial in the behaviour of a marginalised population such as this one. One recent exception was an anthropological study of the work of prostitutes serving migrant Hispanic workers in California, in which it was reported that the women, who were often drug dependent, were sometimes barely conscious of their surroundings because of the intoxication or withdrawal effects of drugs (Magana, 1991). Such women would have sex with many men in quick succession, giving rise to the term 'milk brothers' to describe a phenomenon whereby each man potentially came into contact with the semen of a previous client. Clearly, the potential for spread of HIV from man to man in that situation is high.

Studies of prostitutes or their clients are often criticised on the basis that information collected may have little validity. One recent study which contradicts this view originates from Zimbabwe in which 100 sex workers and 100 clients were interviewed (Wilson et al., 1989). There was consistent agreement on information supplied by prostitute and customer concerning the last paid sex act, suggesting that sex workers' accounts of their behaviour with clients are valid. This study also took account of ethnographic and psychological factors. Not surprisingly, divorce and financial need, often to support children, were the commonest reasons for women entering prostitution. Half the clients were drunk during the last reported sex act and half the prostitutes reported always, or often, being drunk when with a client, factors which are likely to have an important influence on safer sex practices. Furthermore, although often poorly organised, it was suggested that close friendship ties between several pairs of sex workers may have been an important source of motivation for health education and consistent use of condoms.

Male prostitutes constitute a group with specific problems relating to the nature of the sexual act and the degree of control over sexual activity with clients. Their sexual orientation is variable; in the West, the majority are self-identified as homosexual or bisexual (Tomlinson et al., 1991) whereas, in developing countries such as Thailand, greater numbers of heterosexuals may be involved for economic reasons. Male prostitution is illegal in most countries of the world which has the result of making it more clandestine and open to exploitation and less amenable to preventive efforts against spread of STDs and HIV. In the only study of its kind in Great Britain, 47 per cent of a sample of male sex workers enlisted for screening at a central London clinic had evidence of an STD (Tomlinson et al., 1991). In Amsterdam, similar work with 50 men who were prostitutes working from brothels or prostitutes visiting an STD clinic revealed a history of frequent venereal infections. Seroprevalence of HIV was 12.5 per cent (Coutinho, van Andel & Rijsdijk, 1988).

Study of male prostitutes highlights important differences between commercial and private sex with respect to the psychological factors operating in the sexual encounter, particularly in the degree of control held by respective partners. There is now good evidence that personalised models for developing skills and resources aimed at risk reduction among gay men do not hold for male sex workers. In a study of 32 male prostitutes working in Glasgow, Scotland, Bloor et al. (1992) have emphasised the difficulties inherent to a situation in which the sexual demands may be ambiguous and the agenda lies largely with the client. It was reported that male prostitutes who were most in control and least likely to engage in unprotected sex were those who, like their female counterparts, were able to make explicit to the client exactly which services were being offered and which were not for sale, and negotiate the price. Nevertheless, ultimate control of the sexual encounter by the prostitute may be impossible, and the chances of sexual assault remain relatively high for both male and female sex workers alike (Bloor et al., 1992).

The role of clinics for sexually transmitted diseases

People who attend clinics for STDs are often the most sexually active and are an important target for prevention against HIV infection (Kreiss, Carael & Meheus, 1988), particularly heterosexuals in poor inner city areas who face a serious threat of a future epidemic. Psychological factors are important in determining whether patients will attend for review after their first clinic visit. Hammond, Maw and Mulholland (1989) reported that abnormal scores on the Eysenck Personality Inventory could predict poor attendance for review appointments. Simply educating patients to return without considering psychological and social factors, has little impact (Bewley, 1988). There is good evidence that psychological problems are correlated with established risk factors for recurrent genital infections, such as more partners and previous infections (Ross, 1987), which, in turn, has implications for control of HIV infection.

By various criteria, between 30 and 40 per cent of attenders at STD clinics have significant psychiatric problems (Pedder & Goldberg, 1970, Catalan et al., 1981, Ikkos et al., 1987, Barczak et al., 1988). Besides general psychological distress, difficulties are encountered in the context of the service, such as psychosomatic complaints focused on the genitalia (Woodward, 1981), general hypochondriasis (Ross, 1987), venereophobia (Oates & Gomez, 1984) and sexual problems (Catalan et al., 1981). Psychiatric status may even influence recurrence of chronic viral infections such as genital herpes (Goldmeier & Johnson, 1982). Although the role of psychiatrists in an STD clinic has been studied in one small project (Bhanji & Mahony, 1978), there has been no attempt to assess the ability of the venereologist to recognise and manage psychological problems in clinic attenders. Detection and treatment of psychological problems in this population could have important implications for preventing spread of infection, including HIV.

Conclusions

Studies of the sexual behaviour of general populations held little salience for funding bodies prior to the appearance of AIDS. Even today, large-scale surveys are fraught with methodological pitfalls and are rarely undertaken. Information on the sexual behaviour of the wider community is crucial if we are to place in context work on particular groups such as gay men. Work on prevention of spread of HIV has concentrated largely on increasing knowledge about HIV, changing attitudes towards the infection and attempting to reduce unsafe sexual practices. Less work has focused on the important mental health factors which may intervene on the pathway to safer sex practices. From what is known, it would appear that psychiatric problems and use of alcohol and drugs are predictive of a higher frequency of risky sex in young people, be they homosexual or heterosexual. It also appears that increasing knowledge will not in itself lead to a change in behaviour. Rather, attention must be paid to altering mental health variables which may intervene in the process. The factors implicated in a return to unsafe sexual practices have received most study in cohorts of gay men. Not surprisingly, many of the factors which predict unsafe sex also predict a relapse to unsafe sex in those who may have formerly changed their behaviour. However, one reason which is given by men in many studies is the belief that safer sex is less important in primary or monogamous relationships. Unfortunately, the exclusivity of such relationships may break down, exposing either partner to risk of infection if safer sex is abandoned.

Sex workers constitute a particular group with a potential for spread of HIV. However, at least in Western populations, prostitutes appear to be at greatest risk from their private partners or from drug use. The greatest risk to clients would seem to come from sex workers who use drugs. The dilemmas for male prostitutes exemplify the complexities involved in the differential power relationships in sexual encounters, and the difficulties that arise when sexual demands are unclear or where one partner has little ability to control the encounter. There is evidence that psychological factors are also important in the treatment and prevention of STDs which has obvious implications for prevention of AIDS.

CHAPTER SEVEN

ILLICIT DRUG USE AND HIV INFECTION

The association between intravenous drug use and spread of HIV infection is well established in the public and scientific mind. Intravenous drug users (IVDU), however, are much less well organised socially or politically to seek appropriate treatment and resist prejudice than are other groups. Despite increasingly positive approaches to the management of drug use, they remain a singularly unpopular minority. Prevalence of HIV infection in IVDUs may vary widely, even between adjacent geographical areas, and depends on local patterns of needle and syringe sharing and on the mobility of users (Brettle, 1987). Nevertheless, they comprise the fastest growing group of people with AIDS in developed countries. Between 1985 and 1989 the proportion of injecting drug users among people with newly diagnosed AIDS in Europe rose from 15 to 36 per cent, with figures as high as 50 per cent in some regions (Strang, 1991). In New York, for some time, the incidence of new cases of AIDS has been greater in drug users than in homosexual men (Dole, 1989). Up to one-quarter of seropositive drug users on the west coast of the United States also carry antibodies against human T-lymphotropic virus types I and II (Page et al., 1990). These additional viruses appear to worsen the overall prognosis with those who are doubly infected being three times more likely to die over a defined follow-up period. At least one-third of patients in Scotland are women whose infection arises from drug abuse or sexual contact with users (Brettle, 1987). Women face particular difficulties related to economic dependence, pregnancy and child care (Bradbeer, 1989, Selwyn et al., 1989), and their needs are discussed further in Chapter 8. IVDUs have high lifetime rates of sexually transmitted diseases, and sexual transmission of HIV from IV drug users to sexual partners who do not use drugs may be a major route of spread to the wider population (Moss, 1987; Ross et al., 1991).

Legislation against drugs

Despite world-wide efforts against the use of opiates, stimulants, solvents, some classes of tranquillisers and other drugs such as cannabis, abuse of substances has escalated throughout the second half of this century. Although legislation to control the use of opium had been enacted in the United Kingdom in the nineteenth century, governmental regulation of a range of drugs of dependence was first introduced in 1920. Doctors continued, however, to have the power to prescribe controlled drugs even to drug abusers if it was deemed necessary. Increasing drug abuse, and excessive prescribing by a small number of British doctors in the 1960s, led to sharp legal restrictions on the prescribing of heroin and cocaine to special settings (Ministry of Health & Scottish Home & Health Dept, 1965). Some countries in Europe, such as the Netherlands, have attempted to deal with substance abuse by regarding it as primarily a problem of social wellbeing rather than as a criminal matter (Engelsman, 1991). Criminal law is applied in such a way as to decrease the supply of drugs rather than to punish their use. Even the sale of small quantities of cannabis is regarded tolerantly by the police in an attempt to limit underground activity. This less restrictive legal approach is combined with an active, outreach community programme of treatment and education. It is claimed that strategies such as these lead to much less interest in the use of drugs by Dutch youth (Engelsman, 1991). In other countries of Europe, such as Switzerland, there have been experiments wherein drug use is tolerated in demarcated areas to counteract the underworld pattern of use of adulterated substances, criminal activity to enable purchase of drugs at black-market prices, and the sharing of injecting equipment. This type of initiative has had only limited success, however, perhaps as a result of isolation. Greater tolerance of drug use in one region without change in neighbouring regions may simply act as a magnet to attract further problem users to the country carrying out the experiment. Some would go further in suggesting much wider decriminalisation, albeit with some form of State control on sales and distribution (Anon, 1991). Whatever the answer, current criminal law is doing little to stem the flow of drugs and underground use continues to promote transmission of HIV.

Enormous economic forces behind the sales of illicit drugs in the West will ensure that expansion continues.

It is important to emphasise that patterns of substance use are not static. Although, overall use appears to be increasing steadily in most countries of the world, epidemics of specific drug use come and go and are often fundamentally altered by availability of particular substances and local fashions. The inhalation of solvents which was very prevalent among adolescents in Britain during the 1970s, declined in popularity during the 1980s but seems once again to be on the increase. The almost universal injection of heroin which occurred in the 1960s and 1970s has altered through the 1980s, with increasing popularity of inhalation (Strang et al., 1992).

Drug users frequently abuse several different types of substances. In one recent study conducted in the north-west of England, it was found that 90 per cent were polydrug users and 28 per cent were using the tranquillising drug temazepam. One-third of all polydrug users had habitually used more than three drugs in addition to their preferred drug in the previous year. Use of temazepam and extensive polydrug use were associated with sharing injecting equipment and with risky sexual behaviour (Klee et al., 1990). Viewed positively, changing patterns such as these provide opportunities for creative strategies for intervention (Strang, 1991).

Changes in care of drug users

In most Western countries the philosophy of care of drug users has altered profoundly. Although abstinence from drugs and prevention of drug use remains a priority, the emphasis has shifted towards harm reduction and the containment of infection. HIV is regarded as a greater threat to public and individual health than drug misuse. 'Harm minimisation', the catchword of the 1980s, refers to treatment approaches which reduce the harm associated with particular drug use, usually injection. A narrow focus on abstinence is regarded as unrealistic (Brettle, 1987). Prevention of injection and education of users away from injection, towards oral drug use, however, remains crucial.

During the last five years major efforts have been made in Western countries to reach IVDUs in the community with education about safer injecting and safer sex, and the supply of needles and syringes. Professionals, trained in the psychological and social management of drug use, are based in teams directly in the community and develop outreach programmes to drug users wherever they live or congregate. Community drug teams have become a model for care in Europe and North America. They usually work in close liaison with clinic based drug management and HIV services. Problems may arise if there is no doctor in the team, as primary medical care and the prescribing of opiate substitutes can be an important component of the work. In some services, this has been circumvented by close liaison with local primary care physicians who are prepared to treat and prescribe or by attaching a part-time doctor to the team to carry out these roles. Unfortunately, family physicians are often reluctant to become involved with drug users, particularly with IVDUs whom they regard as manipulative and dishonest in their pursuit of prescribed psychoactive drugs. In Britain, there have been several surveys of the attitudes of family doctors to, and their work with, drug users (Glanz, 1986*a*,*b*; King, 1989*a*; Rhodes et al., 1989; Abed & Neira-Munoz, 1990). The evidence suggests that they are not welcomed by general practitioners and are considered unrewarding to treat (see Chapter 9). This reluctance stems from inadequate knowledge about addiction and available management options on the one hand, and inadequate back up from specialist services on the other. Bell, Cohen & Cremona (1990) in a survey of family physicians in inner London reported that three out of four doctors had been consulted by a drug user in the preceding 4 weeks. Evidence from this same survey, however, suggested that medical education on management of drug dependence was inadequate, with only 25 per cent of GPs able to recollect any undergraduate teaching in this field, although 26 per cent had received educational input during postgraduate, vocational training. 35 per cent considered that further training would increase their inclination to deal with the problem, and 27 per cent expressed an interest in further education by the use of small educational groups.

Although many countries lack explicit public health targets for the care of drug users (Strang, 1991), others such as the United States and Britain have published specific recommendations. A report entitled 'Healthy People 2000' recommends that, by the turn of the millennium, 90 per cent of American cities should have developed outreach programmes to deliver HIV risk reduction education to drug users, and that at least 75 per cent of primary care providers should be screening their patients for alcohol and other drug problems, and providing counselling and referral as needed (Presidential Commission on the Human Immunodeficiency Virus Epidemic, 1988). In Britain, a recent government White Paper entitled 'The

Health of the Nation' cites HIV and AIDS as one of five key areas in a strategy to prevent disease and promote better health (Department of Health, 1992). A risk factor target set in the drug use field is 'to reduce the percentage of injecting drug misusers who report sharing equipment in the previous 4 weeks from 20 per cent in 1990 to no more than 10 per cent by 1997 and no more than 5 per cent by 2000.' Although one may argue about the utility of health targets such as this, at least they provide an impetus for research and prevention efforts.

Needle and syringe exchanges

Although a policy of supplying syringes had been undertaken in Britain in the 1960s and 1970s when injectable drugs were prescribed, this practice had all but disappeared with the move to oral methadone (Stimson, 1989). After reports from Edinburgh in 1986 indicated that a high prevalence of HIV in IVDUs was due to sharing, fostered by a lack of syringes and needles, a large expansion in exchange schemes occurred. However, evidence that drug users share injecting equipment because they have difficulty obtaining them, is contradictory. While needles and syringes were sold in Italian pharmacies for some time, HIV prevalence in drug users in that country continued to indicate high levels of sharing (Moss, 1987, Stimson, 1989).

Evidence that needle and syringe exchange programmes prevent spread of HIV is patchy and unconvincing. Evaluation is difficult because of the anonymous ways in which exchanges operate. Many programmes have been evaluated on the basis of return rates for used equipment or reported changes in behaviour when the ultimate test of efficacy rests on whether such schemes have an impact on the rate of spread of HIV in drug using communities. Sharing may persist with trusted friends or sexual partners, among people introduced to drugs for the first time, in prisons, or when 'scoring' from dealers (Stimson, 1989). Nevertheless, in some countries, at least there is more hopeful evidence. On the basis of data on follow-up of users of Sweden's first syringe exchange programme established in 1986, it would appear that early instigation of the programme prevented an epidemic of HIV in the population despite the presence of the virus in that country for more than ten years among homosexual men and six years among drug users (Ljungberg & Christensson, 1991). This is encouraging, when so much evidence for exchange programmes is equivocal, at least with regard to prevention of spread of infection.

Changing the behaviour of drug users

The behaviour of injecting drug users depends to a significant degree on the type of drugs used. In a recent English study comparing amphetamine and heroin users, it was reported that amphetamine users were more socially outgoing, considered that the drug raised their interest in sex and reported more frequent and more casual sex. Although similar levels of sharing occurred in each group, the potential for sexual spread in amphetamine users is clearly of concern (Klee, 1991). There is now a considerable body of research of this type which demonstrates that the nature of the drug used may have a considerable effect on the social relations of drug users and the likelihood of sharing or increased sexual activity (Friedman, Des Jarlais & Sterk, 1990).

The public and the media unfortunately see only the failures of drug treatment programmes. Popular views of drug users as resistant to change in terms of drug use or sexual behaviour do not hold up to examination. In a recent Italian study, 189 injecting drug users participated in a programme consisting of an audiovisual presentation before, and after, HIV testing, as well as receiving individual counselling. Syringe sharing decreased from 35 per cent at initial contact to 12 per cent after six months. Drug users taking part in continuous methadone treatment were less likely to engage in high risk drug-injecting practices than the others. Although sexual behaviour proved more resistant to change, condom use in risky situations increased from 49 per cent to 70 per cent. Whether people are able to recognise a so-called risky situation, however, is very doubtful (Martin et al., 1990).

Audits of outreach programmes which aim to supply information and provide testing for street users in the United States have demonstrated that moderate change in behaviour is possible. Neaigus et al. (1990) interviewed 276 drug users recruited on the streets and followed up 121 (44 per cent) of them a mean of 4.5 months later (Neaigus et al., 1990). Such a large drop-out rate after a relatively short follow-up period is not surprising in this population, but, nevertheless, limits the conclusions. Although significant risk reduction occurred in many drug and sexual risk behaviours, use of bleach showed little change, and more than half of the subjects continued to engage in risky sexual practices. Those who injected less often or were enrolled in drug abuse treatment programmes were more likely to stop high risk drug injecting. Subjects, who at first interview engaged in less frequent unprotected sex, or who had had sex with someone with AIDS, were more likely to stop high risk sexual behaviour. The majority of subjects at low risk at intake maintained low risk behaviour. Thus the authors concluded that educational interventions were most successful among those drug users already engaging in lower levels of risk behaviour and that more effective methods for those whose level of risk behaviour is greater might involve peer pressure and the provision of cleaning materials such as bleach, rather than simply providing information on sterile techniques.

Peer pressure has proved very successful in North America in reducing risky sexual behaviour among gay men. A recent trial of behaviour change carried out among gay men in three small cities in the United States engaged already known, trusted and popular people in the population to serve as 'risk-reduction endorsers' (Kelly et al., 1991). There are natural opinion leaders within any community who may be reliably identified and recruited to participate in peer behaviour change efforts. Although ex-drug users often take a carer role in community drug programmes, users actually living with and relating daily to other drug users may be more successful in disseminating risk reduction behaviour changes.

Evidence that up to 70 per cent of people who experiment with injectable drugs for the first time share equipment (Hart et al., 1989) makes it plain that education to prevent sharing needs to be addressed to young people throughout the community and not simply to current users. There is some recent evidence that this may be having an effect, or that fashions are changing, at least in some areas. In a study of 400 heroin users in London who were interviewed by trained peers, it was reported in a year-by-year analysis of first drug use from the 1950s to the 1990s that 'chasing the dragon', or inhaling heroin after heating it on tinfoil, had become a much more common route of initiation (Strang et al., 1992). Up to the 1970s, only a minority of users inhaled heroin in this manner, by 1981, more than half of initiations were by 'chasing' and, after 1988, over 90% of initiations were conducted in this manner. Although this route of administration may have led to an expansion in the use of heroin, it may explain lower rates of HIV infection. In Scottish and in many Italian cities, however, heroin use appears to continue largely by injection.

Drug use in prisons

Prevalence of HIV in prisoners varies enormously between countries depending on the nature of the prison system, policies on imprisonment of apprehended drug users, methods of surveillance, and the level of drug use in the prison population. For example, in British prisons, HIV antibody testing is only carried out with the informed consent of the prisoner. Routine or anonymous testing does not occur. Many countries, including the United Kingdom, lack data on prevalence of HIV in prisoners, citing reasons of confidentiality for so doing (Harding, 1987). However, data collected in the mid- to late 1980s in several European countries, including Italy and Spain, indicate that rates of seropositivity among prisoners may be as high as 16 to 26 per cent (Harding, 1987, 1990). Rates among prisoners in other countries of the world have been estimated at 17 per cent in Argentina, 18 per cent Brazil, up to 15 per cent in United States, but only 1.4 per cent in Australia (Brewer & Derrickson, 1992)

It has been estimated that between 3400 and 5400 prisoners in Britain's jails were dependent on illicit drugs before entering the prison system (Maden et al., 1991). This represents approximately 10 per cent of the prison population. A report from Scotland of interviews with 559 unselected prisoners revealed that 27.5 per cent had used IV drugs before imprisonment, more than half of whom admitted shared injecting equipment (Power et al., 1992). Other work around the world indicates that between 25 and 30 per cent of prisoners are regular users of opiate drugs before incarceration (Harding, 1987). Drug use appears to continue during the period of incarceration. Carvell and Hart (1990) have estimated that about two-thirds of drug users will inject drugs while in prison, over half of whom will share equipment. In their study, undertaken in 1989, they interviewed 42 male and 8 female, self-selected drug users attending a treatment centre, all of whom had been in prison, on average for 21 months, in the preceding 7 years. One woman and four men were also sexually active while in custody, with a mean of seven partners. Power et al. (1992) in their study of Scottish prisoners reported that almost 8 per cent used IV drugs while in prison, three-quarters of whom shared equipment. About half of those who shared, however, used some form of sterilisation procedure.

It takes little imagination to realise that, by its restrictive nature, the prison environment must lead to extensive sharing of needles and syringes (Prison Reform Trust, 1988). Although of varying methodology and quality, other studies have reached similar conclusions for British prisons (Hart et al., 1989; Dye & Isaacs, 1991). The picture in the United States appears to be even more serious with steep rises in prevalence of HIV infection in institutions through the mid- to late 1980s and estimates that as many as 70 per cent of inmates of urban prisons may be seropositive

(Valdiserri, Harl & Chambliss, 1988) Although not all drug use in prison entails injection of drugs, when sharing does occur, it is extensive with up to 100 people using one needle (Kennedy et al., 1991).

Another cultural phenomenon common in many prisons which involves needles, and carries a potential for spread of HIV infection, is the custom of tattooing. Prison tattooing is a social activity and involves considerable sharing of needles with a lack of resources for sterilisation, not seen associated with tattooing in the community. It is especially common in institutions for young offenders when a variety of improvised, often dirty equipment is employed (Curran, McHugh & Mooney, 1989).

Not only is drug use and associated sharing of equipment highly likely in many prison settings, but little in the way of treatment is offered to drug users who find themselves in custody. Of 56 injecting drug users interviewed in Scotland who had been recently in custody, 51 (91 per cent) claimed that they had received no treatment for their substance abuse, despite prison authorities awareness of the problem in 46 of the 51 cases. Women were more likely to be offered withdrawal programmes than men (Kennedy et al., 1991) which may be a result of pilot schemes to treat drug dependence established in one of Britain's prisons for women in 1987 (Madden, Swinton & Gunn, 1990). Further discussion of the needs of women prisoners is considered in Chapter 8. This apparent lack of facility in prisons for controlled withdrawal not only encourages continued use and sharing of equipment but also wastes an opportunity to provide education and prevention. Recent guidelines from the English Prison Medical Service now recommend that a detoxification programme with oral methadone should be offered routinely to all new prisoners with opiate addiction.

Prison authorities vary widely in their reaction to seropositive prisoners. In some countries, prisoners are segregated while, in others, such as Austria and Switzerland, treatment is liberal and condoms are distributed. One-quarter of prison institutions across Europe in the late 1980s were reported to have rulings on the segregation of seropositive prisoners (Harding, 1990), despite lack of evidence that segregation of such prisoners is helpful, except in the most exceptional circumstances (Farrell & Strang, 1991). Segregation implies that those who are not segregated are not infected. Prisoners who are known to be HIV antibody positive are likely to receive verbal or physical expressions of hostility from other prisoners, ranging from verbal suggestions or threats to extreme cases where fires are set in the prisoner's cell (Curran et al., 1989). A survey in the 1980s showed that, although prisoners were knowledgeable about routes of transmission of

HIV, they were reluctant to share any prison facility with fellow prisoners who were seropositive (Curran et al., 1989). Fortunately, educational programmes about HIV infection for staff and prisoners in British prisons have been developed and made available, and may go some way to ameliorate this situation. Explicit advice contained in the programmes, however, has not always gone without opposition from prison authorities (Curran, personal communication). Similarly, in the United States, nearly all prison facilities provide AIDS-specific education, although some prison authorities pitched the level of their education at too low a level. Inmates' knowledge is, in fact, comparable with that of the US adult population (Brewer & Derrickson, 1992).

Although it is often assumed that sexual behaviour occurs between prisoners, research to substantiate this belief is difficult to conduct. Reports vary depending on the type and sensitivity of the questions asked. Some reports indicate that between 20 and 30 per cent of long-term male prisoners in Britain may have sex with other men while incarcerated (Prison Reform Trust, 1988). In others, it is claimed that rates are very low (Power et al., 1991). Results depend greatly on the form of the research. Careful, well-designed enquiry which avoids embarrassingly direct questioning or technical language indicates that homosexual behaviour between men who are fundamentally heterosexual in orientation is common in prisons. Furthermore, coercive sexual activity, even frank assault, occurs regularly but is often hidden and denied through fear of stigma, or because of a threat of further victimisation (King, 1992*a*).

In addition to the need for more determined efforts to protect prisoners against victimisation, arguments have been advanced for the provision of condoms and clean needles and syringes (Harding, 1990). It must be noted, however, that condoms are not always welcomed by prisoners, their availability being regarded as an accusation of homosexual behaviour. The only certain alternative to the provision of condoms is enforced isolation, and close supervision of prisoners during social intermingling (McMillan, 1988), which would be intolerable. An environment in which sharing of needles and syringes is relatively common, and anal sex no less so, is potentially explosive in terms of HIV spread. Arguments against condom distribution in prisons are based on a fear that to do so would promote sexual activity, which is technically illegal, or a concern that they might be used as weapons or to smuggle drugs. Fine points on the illegality of homosexual activity in prisons can even inhibit education on safer sex (Harding, 1990). Unfortunately, there seems little likelihood of condoms, needles or syringes being made available to inmates of United States prisons at least in the near future (Brewer & Derrickson, 1992). Meanwhile, HIV transmission goes on, more prisoners become infected, and once out of prison transmission continues to their partners and children.

Drug use and prostitution

Prostitution is the only economic resource for many drug users. HIV antibody prevalence is very variable among female prostitutes, varying with geographical region between 0 and 44 per cent, higher rates being found in larger inner cities (Magana, 1991). AIDS in Thailand is expanding rapidly among an estimated 100 000 IV drug users and 500 000 prostitutes. In 1989, it was estimated that 700 people seroconverted each month, 86 per cent of whom had injected drugs (Anderson, 1990). Female drug users in parts of the USA are frequently heavily dependent on injected drugs. Although having sex with multiple clients, condom usage may be discouraged out of concern that they will be regarded as diseased or from fear that condoms would be considered incriminating evidence should they be stopped by police (Magana, 1991).

Up to 150 male prostitutes, mostly hard drug users, solicit daily on the streets of Amsterdam (Van den Hoek, Van Haastrecht & Coutinho, 1991). In a study of 449 male drug users in Holland, 343 of whom injected drugs, 88 (20 per cent) reported engaging in prostitution, although no evidence was found to suggest that male prostitution in itself contributed to the risk of HIV infection (Van den Hoek et al., 1991). Whether it contributed to the risk in the clients of such men is an open question. In Italy, 57 male, transvestite prostitutes, who were also drug users, underwent HIV antibody testing and took part in an interview about their drug use and sexual behaviours (Gattari et al., 1992). The overall prevalence of HIV antibody was 74 per cent. HIV prevalence increased with the duration of drug use, rising from 48 per cent for less than two years' use, to 64 per cent for two to four years, and 100 per cent for more than four years. Prevalence of HIV antibody was higher among those who reported injecting drugs or who reported needle sharing. Higher prevalence was also related to the number of partners in the last year, but numbers of partners were very high across the whole group. Not using condoms was also related to higher HIV prevalence. With some of the men reporting over 1500 clients per year, this group presents a major potential for spread and further educational outreach efforts are essential. The issue of drug use and sexual behaviour, including prostitution, is also discussed in Chapters 6 and 8.

Psychiatric disorders in drug users

Whether the care of drug users should be the responsibility of medicine, or more particularly of psychiatry, remains unresolved. Repetitious debate over social versus medical models of drug dependence, and whether certain personality types predispose to drug use, has not been universally helpful. In the opinion of some, the medical profession has abdicated its role with drug users by abandoning their care to other professionals, mainly those in the social services (Dole, 1989). There is considerable evidence, however, that they are not welcomed by doctors and are considered unrewarding to treat (Glanz, 1986*a*,*b*; King, 1989*a*). The majority of users do not conform to the 'junkie' stereotype of the chaotic user with many psychological and social problems, but lead a stable existence usually on a contract of continuing treatment. Careful studies using matched populations have demonstrated that drug users are no more likely than other groups to suffer psychiatric disorder (Neville, McKellican & Foster, 1988), although there is often a history of dishonest or violent behaviour. For most psychiatrists, contact with drug users will usually arise when major psychiatric problems such as psychotic and confusional states occur, usually as a consequence of the drug use itself. When chaotic drug use, HIV infection and neuropsychiatric complications coincide, major difficulties for the liaison psychiatrist are likely to ensue. Interpretation of deficits on cognitive testing must take account of prior drug abuse which may have caused impairment on psychomotor tasks well before infection with HIV (Egan et al., 1990). Thus, although impairment on neuropsychological testing may not herald the onset of HIV encephalopathy, it may none the less damage an individual's ability to cope with the stress of the illness. Cognitive impairment in HIV infection is considered more fully in Chapter 5. Bizarre, or otherwise unexplained, psychological symptoms, particularly in inpatients, may also be due to continued drug use, with supplies provided by visitors to the ward. Thus, judicious urine screens for illicit psychoactive drugs should become established practice on wards whenever such behaviour is suspected.

Provision of drug-related and HIV medical services at the same site by the same doctors appears to provide the most efficient service for drug users with HIV, but has yet to be systematically evaluated (Brettle, 1990). If HIV antibody testing, HIV care and drug management are provided in the same service, IVDUs may be more likely to take up antibody testing, change behaviours and attend more regularly for HIV management. As a group, they are not particularly consistent attenders to hospital HIV services which are divorced from drug management. Appropriate placement of drug users ill with AIDS who may, hitherto, have lived in inadequate housing or on the streets, poses enormous problems for carers. Patients may either reject offers of public housing or masquerade as seropositive in order to qualify for special consideration in obtaining such accommodation. Perhaps the most successful social and psychological support can be provided by specialised counsellors who have formerly used drugs themselves.

Conclusions

Use of illicit drugs continues to expand in many countries, propelled by a powerful, economic underworld. Valuable revenues stem from the production and exportation of substances which are illegal to possess, or take, in most Western countries, and several developing countries in the world stand to benefit from the much needed foreign currency which accrues from the trade. Efforts to criminalise drug-taking behaviour have done little to prevent its spread but have done much to force drug use underground and promote the spread of HIV infection. However, limited efforts to decriminalise drug use in certain parts of the world have met with varying degrees of success and require substantial back-up with counselling and educational resources. Rates of HIV seroprevalence among drug users vary widely across the world, but explosive epidemics have occurred in countries such as Thailand. Behaviour change among drug users depends as much on psychological and social factors as on knowledge about HIV infection itself. The nature of the drugs taken may profoundly alter the chances of sharing needles and syringes or the occurrence of risky sexual behaviour. HIV infection in prisons is most intimately related to drug use both within and without the prison walls, but is also related to same sex encounters between prisoners, the extent of which may have been underestimated in some surveys. Mental health professionals who do not specialise in the drug field have little to do with the care of users unless major psychiatric difficulties supervene. For carers of people with AIDS, the chaotic lifestyle of some drug users can combine with personality, psychological and cognitive difficulties to make these patients among the most difficult to treat. An integrated service which is able to deliver medical, psychiatric and drug-related care on the same site is the ideal for drug users with HIV disease.

CHAPTER EIGHT

SPECIAL GROUPS

In Western countries, three groups of people with particular concerns relating to HIV infection can be distinguished, and are most readily considered in their own right. In this chapter, I will explore the psychological needs and difficulties of women, children, and people who have contracted HIV through transfusion of contaminated blood products.

Women with HIV infection

The World Health Organisation (WHO) has reported that during the first decade of the AIDS pandemic, about 500 000 cases of AIDS in women and children occurred, much of which went unrecognised. During the 1990s, the WHO estimates that the infection will kill at least an additional three million women and children world-wide (Chin, 1990). Women are contributing about one-third of new cases of HIV infection in Scotland and one-sixth in England, Wales and Northern Ireland (Norman et al., 1990). AIDS has become the leading cause of death for young women, and infant mortality may be as much as 30 per cent higher than expected, in major cities in North and South America, Western Europe and sub-Saharan Africa (Chin, 1990). Furthermore, several million uninfected children will be orphaned because a large proportion of HIV-infected mothers will die of AIDS.

Interest in the specific psychological and behavioural problems related to women with HIV infection was slow to develop. Initial concern focused on the risks of maternal infection, how infected women might be identified, and how they might be discouraged from becoming pregnant (Bayer, 1990). Prostitutes were often identified as possible infectious agents for their male clients, often with little empirical evidence to confirm the assumption. In the West, the social impact of HIV on women was considered insignificant compared to that of gay men. Volunteer programmes originated mainly from the gay community and AIDS was perceived as a 'gay male disease' by many researchers (Worth, 1990). Despite recent attention such as the dedication of World AIDS Day in 1990 to women infected with HIV, it is still not completely clear why the effects on women were for so long ignored. Even within the considerable body of research on the behavioural factors in HIV infection, there has been a conspicuous lack of attention to specific issues for women (Sherr & Strong, 1992).

Decision-making about heterosexual relations and child bearing for women is inextricably linked to their socioeconomic standing, self-esteem and dependency relationships with men (Sherr, 1991). It is often assumed that women are able to control the sexual encounter. In fact, the responsibility for use of either fertility control or prevention of infection is an area of considerable difficulty for many women. Women who carry condoms and suggest that they are used may be regarded as 'fast' or 'easy'. Prostitutes may be induced to forego use of condoms for greater monetary reward. Infected women who wish to avoid penetrative sex to protect their partner may be unable to negotiate this successfully (Worth, 1990). When women are asked directly about these issues, it is clear that they perceive themselves as relatively powerless in many sexual encounters or relationships (Sherr & Strong, 1992) and, even if they are open about their serostatus, they find that their partners take little action to protect themselves and insist on intercourse without condoms (Brown & Rundell, 1990; Mellers, J., personal communication). One graphic example of these difficulties for women stems from a recent prospective study of counselling and educational interventions for couples discordant for HIV infection in Rwanda (Allen et al., 1992). Condoms were used more consistently by discordant couples when the *man* was the HIV negative partner. It would appear that the effectiveness of any programme promoting condom use depends on its acceptance by the male partner. Furthermore, in all of the discordant couples in which the HIV seronegative partner seroconverted during the time of the study, the man was reported to drink alcohol regularly.

The risk of transmission of HIV from mother to baby *in utero* is in the order of 15 per cent in Western countries providing good obstetric care. The risk is higher in developing countries, where the prevalence of genital ulceration, with its potential for intrapartum transmission, is higher. These issues are discussed in greater detail later in this chapter in a consideration of HIV infection in children. Although it was often assumed that a high proportion of women who found themselves infected with HIV would wish to terminate their pregnancy for fear of risk to the baby, or on the assumption of a limited lifespan in which to care for a child, recent evidence does not bear this out. A desire to have a baby may override all other considerations. Johnstone et al. (1990) studied decisions taken regarding the continuation of pregnancy by 163 women in Scotland who had either used intravenous drugs or had been the partner of an infected drug user. Although this group of women had a high rate of induced abortion overall, there was little difference with regard to HIV status. Finding that they were HIV seropositive during pregnancy did little to alter the women's original intention. Many women were influenced by their own lack of clinical illness, and by recent reports in the media that the risks to the foetus were lower than previously estimated. Similar controlled comparisons in the United States had already drawn comparable conclusions, namely that socio-economic considerations were more salient than infection with HIV in determining a woman's decision to request termination. Selwyn et al. (1989) reported that the rate of elective abortion among seronegative and seropositive women were very similar at 44 and 50 per cent, respectively. Pregnancy-related factors were more predictive of termination. These factors were a prior elective abortion, a negative emotional reaction to the pregnancy and whether the pregnancy was unplanned.

Thus, knowledge of HIV status has little impact on reproductive decisions. Other psychological and social factors related to the pregnancy appear to be of greater importance. However, this does not mean that counselling about the issues becomes irrelevant. The provision of testing and counselling offers women useful information in making a fully informed reproductive decision, educates them about sexually transmitted diseases, and assists in bringing education to their partners (Landesman, Minkoff & Willoughby, 1989).

Despite these findings, there remains a danger that medical practitioners or nurses who are apprehensive about seropositive women going to term may directly or indirectly influence them to undergo therapeutic abortion. It has even been questioned whether gynaecologists should be prepared to support seropositive women who are determined to proceed with a pregnancy or help those who request advice for infertility (Norman et al.,

1990). Reports of individual, seropositive women who proceed with a pregnancy and experience being treated badly by attending physicians do nothing to lessen the concern (Brown & Rundell, 1990). In more enlightened services when pregnancy is a pressing issue, particularly for couples in which the woman is seronegative, women are advised that unprotected sexual intercourse should be restricted to their time of maximum fertility in mid-cycle. Serial antibody testing is offered throughout the pregnancy and, if seroconversion occurs before 20 weeks, termination may be discussed (Miller et al., 1989*b*). Just as in genetic counselling, all aspects of the infection should be reviewed before any informed decision can be taken. The professional's personal views on the ethical or moral issues regarding pregnancy and HIV should not influence decision-making or management. There is a great need for debate about, and clarification of, issues related to individual and reproductive freedom (Bayer, 1990).

It was only with the development of counselling and educational programmes targeted specifically at women that knowledge about the impact on them of the infection began to increase (Worth, 1990). Psychological reactions in women must be regarded in the context of their cultural and socioeconomic status. Women at most risk for HIV infection are poor, black and belong to socially less favoured groups such as the Hispanic-speaking population of the United States. They are less likely to receive adequate health care (Landesman et al., 1989). Few studies have centred on the psychological issues for infected seropositive women, and even fewer have made controlled comparisons with seronegative women. In a small study in an inner London clinic for women with HIV infection, (Mellers et al., 1991), we carried out structured psychiatric and social assessments on 24 women with HIV infection attending for regular gynaecological surveillance, and on a control group of 13 women attenders without HIV infection. Although rates of formal psychiatric disorder as measured by standardised psychiatric interview were relatively low, and comparable to men with HIV infection assessed by the same standardised psychological rating scales, concern about the social stigma of the infection and the dilemmas relating to sexual behaviour and child bearing were common. Principal psychiatric conditions encountered were depressive disorders and adjustment reactions. Those HIV seropositive women who were in a sexual relationship often had particular difficulties convincing partners who were cognisant of their serostatus to use condoms.

Brown & Rundell (1990) have reported on the first phase of a detailed five-year prospective study of 20 seropositive women who were not drug users. The women had discovered their HIV serostatus as part of the United States Air Force mandatory screening programme initiated in 1986, and were described as more 'representative' of women who acquire the infection through heterosexual intercourse. Over 90 per cent had known the diagnosis for more than 12 months. No direct comparison group was used but data were compared with male Air Force personnel also subjected to mandatory testing. Although 35 per cent were assigned a DSMIIIR Axis I diagnosis, over half of the diagnoses were hypoactive sexual desire disorder. Adjustment disorders were the next most important diagnosis. Suicidal ideas at any time since knowledge of HIV serostatus were uncommon in contrast to the male personnel in which rates of up to 25 per cent were reported. Progression of HIV infection over a one year follow-up was related to psychiatric conditions in only two women and, in each case, this occurred on an organic basis. Curiously, there was little comment in the paper on the impact of mandatory testing for this subject group or on the effect of positive serostatus on the women's future career in the Air Force.

The effects of AIDS on women in special circumstances such as psychiatric care or in prisons have also been studied. Knowledge about AIDS in women under psychiatric care has been studied on the presumption that risk factors, such as intravenous drug abuse, are more prevalent in this population (Aruffo et al., 1990). Eighty women aged between 18 and 40 years who were psychiatric outpatients at a college-affiliated, community psychiatric clinic in Houston, Texas were compared with 80 women matched for race and age attending medical clinics. Almost one-half of each group were black and 50 per cent of the psychiatric patients had a diagnosis of schizophrenia. Non whites had lower scores on overall knowledge about HIV infection than whites in both groups. The psychiatric patients, however, were much less knowledgeable about AIDS than the women in the comparison group. The main difference between the groups was accounted for by the low levels of knowledge of the patients with schizophrenia, which could not be explained on the basis of their cognitive ability. Fourteen per cent of the psychiatric patients used intravenous drugs and 73 per cent were sexually active, yet only 53 per cent knew that condoms help to prevent transmission of HIV. These findings highlight the special education and counselling needs of women with chronic psychiatric disorders.

Perceptions about health, AIDS, and the need for AIDS education were explored among a small group of women prisoners in the United States (Viadro & Earp, 1991). Forty short-term inmates took part in group interviews while 16 women completed a detailed questionnaire. Women expressed concerns about AIDS within prison, sexual activity between inmates, and the institution's policy of maintaining seropositive women within the general prison population. Forty-four per cent of respondents believed that they were likely to be exposed to HIV in prison, 81 per cent considered that AIDS education programmes should discuss lesbian activity and 94 per cent felt that women prisoners should be given an HIV antibody test upon entering prison. These findings are limited by the small and possibly unrepresentative nature of the subjects and by a failure to consider psychological and personality variables. Nevertheless, there is little other information on this special group and it suggests that AIDS education and prevention activities need to be tailored for women in prisons.

Children with HIV infection

The majority of children with HIV infection contract the virus *in utero* from their HIV seropositive mother. Others may have received the virus via transfused blood products. There is also some evidence of a low risk of transmission from breast milk (Bradbeer, 1989). The passage of HIV maternal antibodies across the placenta leads to difficulties in interpreting a positive HIV antibody test in an infant. Clearance of such antibodies is usually complete by 12 months but may take up to 18 months in some children. Thus HIV infection in children should be diagnosed on clinical grounds, by isolation of the virus, by a positive test for p24 antigen or by a positive antibody test in those over two years of age (Mok, 1988). Clearly, the uncertainty as to the origins of antibodies in seropositive infants will persist throughout the first months of life and there is a need not to over-investigate.

The rate of transplacental, intrapartum and postpartum transfer from infected mother to baby was initially considered to be in the order of 30 to 50 per cent (The European Collaborative Study, 1988). More recent work suggests, however, that rates of perinatal transmission are much lower, perhaps in the region of 15 to 30 per cent (Norman et al., 1990). Genital ulceration may predispose to higher rates of transmission at the time of parturition. This is likely to be the reason for higher rates of transmission in developing countries where treatment of sexually transmitted diseases is less comprehensive. There is no definite evidence, at least in Western countries, that babies born to HIV-infected mothers are at increased risk of prematurity or growth retardation (Johnstone et al., 1988), although, clearly, other factors, such as maternal malnutrition and intravenous drug use, may confound the issue.

Children with HIV infection are at risk of considerable morbidity and mortality. Families in which other members are also infected change the dynamics from that of the more familiar situation of other chronic childhood diseases. The mother or father may be ill and unable to care for the child. There follows all the difficulties inherent to the management of infected children at school, nurseries or in full institutional care. Although guidelines have been issued in many countries for the instruction of professionals in institutional and educational settings, fear on the part of other children or their families may continue to pose a problem (Mok, 1988).

There has been much less work on the psychological problems suffered by children with HIV infection. Although HIV infection in young children appears to lead to neurodevelopmental delays, evidence is conflicting and needs to be carefully considered alongside other possible risk factors for the children, such as health of the mother or maternal use of intravenous drugs during pregnancy. One report in which these effects were controlled for was that by Condini et al. (1991) who studied 36 Italian children aged between 18 and 30 months, born to HIV-1 infected mothers. The children, who were in good health, were studied for speech development by matching 18 infected, with 18 non-infected, subjects for age, sex and socioeconomic status. Both HIV infected, and non-infected, children progressed in language acquisition from the second to the third year of age, but infected children had significantly greater word production difficulty, than non-infected children, in the second year of life. Thus it would appear that HIV-1 infection impairs the genesis rather than the later development of language in infected but well children.

The neuropsychological development of 15 HIV-1 seropositive children infected via neonatal blood transfusion was compared with that of a control group of 33 seronegative children who had also received blood transfusions as neonates (Cohen et al., 1991). Two-thirds of the infected children were asymptomatic at the time of enrolment in the study of development. The children were administered two psychological batteries 8 months apart. Although the two serostatus groups did not differ in overall intelligence, even as long as eight years after HIV-1 infection, slight, but significant, group differences were found on school achievement and on tasks that required motor speed, visual scanning, and cognitive flexibility. Further follow-up of this group will be necessary to see whether these slight gaps between the children widen, in the absence of overt HIV disease.

Children in families where the father is haemophiliac, or children who have haemophilia themselves, have also been the subject of study. In a Scottish study, 43 children with haemophilia, aged between 3 and 16 years were matched with control groups of diabetic and normal children. A diabetic group was included to control for chronic illness and to allow an examination on children of the effects specifically related to haemophilia. The study was conducted during a time of intense media coverage about AIDS in Britain when it was expected that the haemophiliac children might have been affected by social hostility or by over-protectiveness from parents. Haemophiliac children were no more disturbed than their diabetic or healthy peers, but there were slightly increased rates of behavioural disturbance in diabetic children aged between three and five years. Although the importance of these results must be tempered by the small numbers, this lack of distress in either haemophiliac or diabetic children was thought to reflect the substantial psychological and social support offered in both clinics.

Transmission of HIV infection by blood products

AIDS was recognised among recipients of blood, or blood products, by early 1983. Up to 12000 people in the United States were infected via transfused blood before screening began (Freidland & Klein, 1987). In the USA, donated blood and plasma was first screened for antibodies to HIV in April 1985, and heat treatment of clotting factors, screening of donors and discouragement of donors who might be at risk, has all but eliminated risk of transmission by this route (Friedland & Klein, 1987).

Haemophilia is a life-threatening, sex-linked, inherited condition for which supportive treatment must be given by replacement of clotting factors VIII or IX. Because many donors contribute to the plasma pool from which these products are obtained, the chances of virus transmission were increased. Until the early 1980s, Britain imported many blood products from the United States, a country in which blood donors are paid for their donation. Financial incentives increase the likelihood that unsuitable donors, such as those who have abused drugs might be included. Seventy to 80 per cent of persons with haemophilia in the US have been infected with the virus. In Britain, rates of infection with the virus were between 6 and 59 per cent, according to the severity of the haemophilia, and the origin of the blood products used (AIDS Group of the UK Haemophilia Centre Directors, 1988). This has had major medico-legal implications and, despite government attempts to compensate patients, led to litigation organised by patient groups, who claimed that the British Government should have acted earlier to screen blood and prevent imports of blood products, particularly from the USA (Dyer, 1989, 1990). In France there has been enormous public concern about blood products, contaminated by HIV, allegedly being distributed for commercial reasons, despite prior knowledge about the contamination. The head of the Blood Transfusion Service in that country together with two other physicians, have stood trial and been convicted for their involvement in the affair.

Although haemophiliac patients who are seropositive do not carry the additional stigma of drug use or homosexuality and are even regarded as 'innocent victims' (Curran et al., 1984), they and their families have been rejected for fear of the disease itself. Fear of contamination is the commonest reason for the marginalisation of adults and children with HIV infection, despite clear evidence from Western (Freidland & Klein, 1987) and African countries (Mann et al., 1986) that even close personal contact presents no risk to other people. Haemophiliac families are aware that their HIV infection occurred as a result of medical treatment and that this may have also occurred throughout their extended family owing to the inherited nature of haemophilia. This has inevitably led to an ambivalence in their relationship with professional staff of haemophilia treatment units. Although the subject of little empirical research, the staff of haemophilia centres have also had to resolve the dilemma of having cared for their patients *and* unwittingly having been instrumental in transmission of the virus (Miller & Harrington, 1989).

Families where the father is haemophiliac will also have the responsibility of telling children, who may themselves be infected, and who may eventually be bereaved of their father and even possibly of their mother. Wives of haemophiliac men have to cope not only with their husbands' worries about health but also with the problems of taking precautions for sex, and the risks inherent to having children by their husbands (Dew, Ragni & Nimorwicz, 1991). Discussion about sex between parents and their adolescent children may have to be more explicit, creating difficulties for both parents and children (Miller & Harrington, 1989). Young haemophiliac men growing up aware of their HIV status face major difficulties in developing and sustaining sexual relationships. Not only do they experience normal adolescent anxieties about sexuality and sexual behaviour but they must consider protecting their partner from their very first sexual encounter. Some master this successfully, while others have greater difficulty.

Mr W. was a 17 year-old, haemophiliac male, nearing completion of high school who was referred because of depressed mood, apathy and poor concentration in his studies. He had been an outgoing boy whose haemophilia had been reasonably well controlled and who had seemed to cope easily with learning of his HIV serostatus 2 years earlier. His family had been more affected and, despite some intensive family work after the diagnosis, the topic of AIDS was rarely discussed. While experiencing heterosexual interests, he had not ventured to have sex because he feared having to discuss his serostatus with a potential partner and that the news of his infection would then spread. He was very embarrassed by his inexperience in sexual matters and became irritated when other boys jokingly implied that his lack of experience with girls must indicate that he was homosexual. Although suspicious that some of his school friends considered that he might be seropositive, he had never been challenged on the subject. On mental state examination, he was moderately depressed with mild difficulties in concentration. He was in good physical health with T-cell counts in the normal range. There were no signs of significant cognitive impairment.

Psychotherapeutic treatment focused on his concerns about sexual development, his difficulties concentrating at school and his ideas for a future career. Antidepressant drugs were not indicated. Over several months he developed a good rapport in individual therapy and was able to discuss his sexual anxieties in some detail. It quickly became apparent that his family's difficulty in talking about the HIV infection had compounded his distress. His apparent ready acceptance of the diagnosis two years earlier had masked a shock and turmoil that had not been fully expressed. His depressed mood lifted and he managed to progress from school to college. Later he began dating girls and when last seen was much less concerned about proposing use of a condom when first attempting sex.

Well before the appearance of HIV it was known that patients with haemophilia were vulnerable to an excess of psychological and social problems, particularly before the introduction of modern treatments (Smit, Rosendaal & Varekamp, 1989). Problems relate to the vagaries of a chronic, sometimes debilitating, lifelong disease. There is anxiety about children, guilt about the genetic transmission of the disease, and isolation from normal peers because of bleeds and consequent disability. However, it must be emphasised that the availability of adequate replacement therapy over the past 20 years has led to considerable improvements in the life expectancy and physical wellbeing of people with haemophilia. A recent study of the relationships, marriage, family life and employment status of 935 Dutch haemophiliacs revealed that they did not differ from the general population in their view of the quality of their own health (Rosendaal et al., 1990). Although, at present, AIDS may have diminished enthusiasm about this field, the results of this study show a positive influence of modern haemophilia treatment on quality of life, and it is against this background that the effects of AIDS must be considered.

There has been much less empirical study of the psychological status of seropositive haemophiliacs than of analogous homosexual men or IV drug users. The haemophiliac population is less easily accessible but allows for more representative sampling. Work on possible neuropsychological impairment in haemophiliac patients with HIV infection or AIDS has been carried out in a few centres and is considered in more detail in Chapter 5 on the neuropsychiatry of HIV infection. In a well-conducted study of 75 haemophiliac men, 31 of whom were HIV positive, Dew, Ragni & Nimorwicz (1990) recently demonstrated that seropositive men have increased levels of depression, anxiety and anger. Associations with depression and anxiety were a personal history of psychiatric distress, a family history of psychiatric illness, lower levels of education, low support from wives, family or friends, a poor sense of mastery, or recent experience of life events involving loss. These data echo those described in Chapter 3 for homosexual men, where perceived social support is an important factor in psychological health. Although cross-sectional in design, the authors claimed that their study demonstrated that overall levels of *past* psychiatric disorder did not differ between HIV positive and negative men, implying that current distress was a reflection of positive serostatus.In a comparison of 37 seropositive, and 36 seronegative, haemophiliac men in England it was also reported that levels of psychological distress, as measured by the Present State Examination, a structured psychiatric interview (Wing, 1974), were higher in the seropositive haemophiliac men (Catalan et al., 1992). Although 84 per cent of the seropositive men in this study were asymptomatic (Centres for Disease Control stages II or III), they were significantly more likely than seronegatives to report negative consequences on their sexual functioning. Although differences between the groups were significant, they were generally low and not altogether different from what would be found in a general outpatient medical population. This finding echoes work with unselected populations of homosexual men with HIV infection (King, 1989*b*). Factors associated with psychological disturbance in the seropositive group were: high levels of hopelessness as measured by standardised rating scale, a psychiatric history, poor social adjustment, and symptomatic HIV disease. At follow-up, 18 months later, all psychological differences between seropositive and seronegative haemophiliac men had disappeared. Only concerns about sexual activity and the possibility of infecting a partner remained significantly different in the seropositive group (Catalan, 1990). Although Catalan speculated that the improvement at 18 months may have been associated with less media coverage than at the outset of the study, or improved medical care for HIV infection in the haemophilia field, the exact reasons for the change remained unclear.

Further information on the problems for haemophiliac men with HIV infection comes from a study in Sweden in which 43 seropositive men were compared with 30 age-matched seronegative haemphiliacs (Blomqvist, Jonsson & Theorell, 1991). A small group of parents of HIV-infected haemophiliac boys were also studied. Although there were methodological problems in this study which limit the significance of the findings, it was reported that the seropositive men were very pessimistic about the future. The reactions of the parents to the news of their child's infection was apparently more devastating than the reactions of the seropositive men to their own infection, demonstrating the extreme stresses that result in families.

The partners of haemophiliac men have also received research attention. Dew et al. (1991) have recently published a study of 37 wives of haemophiliac men for 17 of whom the husband was seropositive. Perhaps surprisingly, levels of emotional distress in the women were very similar to that found in community samples and there was no relationship between psychiatric symptoms and their husband's serostatus or severity of haemophilia. Women who were employed, however, were more likely to show distress, possibly because of the extra burden of work and a concern to do more for their husbands. A number of women had left employment out of concern for their husband's health. Women who perceived themselves to be at high risk for AIDS were more likely to be emotionally distressed, and recent life events involving loss were also important in determining the woman's psychiatric status. Similar findings have been reported by Klimes et al. (1992) in a controlled study of the partners of 17 HIV seropositive and 19 HIV seronegative haemophiliac men, living near a provincial English city. The partners of seropositive men did not suffer more psychological difficulties, as measured by structured interview and rating scales, although levels of psychological symptoms were higher than in comparable community groups. Those women who reported a history of psychiatric or social difficulties were more vulnerable. Interestingly, women suffered more psychological symptoms than their partners, whether or not the man was HIV positive. This may have been due to the burden that some women bear as carers or because women are inherently more likely to admit to emotional difficulties. Although HIV issues affected the sexual relationships of both seropositive and seronegative couples, the relationships of seropositive couples were more adversely affected than those in which the man was seronegative. Somewhat suprisingly, one-third of the women partnered with seronegative men worried about the possibility of catching HIV. These findings, together with the fact that condoms were not used consistently in the seropositive couples, indicate a need for more detailed discussion of sexual issues with such couples. These studies are among the few that have considered heterosexual partners of men with HIV infection. Although the results are somewhat reassuring, confirmation of low levels of morbidity is awaited from larger samples examined prospectively.

Conclusions

Women have particular difficulties relating to HIV infection that were ignored for some time after the appearance of AIDS. Levels of psychiatric morbidity among women with HIV infection appear to be similar to those in analogous male populations, but the emotional and social issues have a different focus. Women appear to be concerned mostly with effects on child bearing and on their ability to control sexual encounters. Women in particular circumstances such as those in prisons may need information tailored to meet their special requirements.

Children with HIV infection have been the focus of studies to determine impairment in neuropsychological development but have been involved less in studies of the emotional impact of the virus on them and their families. The effect of HIV on neurological development in well, seropositive children has not yet been clearly disentangled from the confounding effects of socioeconomic factors, maternal substance use during pregnancy, maternal health and ability to care for the child.

Controlled studies in haemophiliac men demonstrate, perhaps surprisingly, that, although overall levels of psychological distress may be higher in seropositives than seronegatives, they are only moderately raised, and levels of distress in partners and other family members are not particularly elevated. Lifelong medical supervision of many haemophiliacs by specialised units may have gone some way to ameliorate the emotional impact of HIV. The reduced stigma associated with HIV in haemophilia, however, is also likely to be contributory.

CHAPTER NINE

HEALTH PROFESSIONALS AND ASSOCIATED CARE GIVERS

Just as AIDS has generated controversy in society, its appearance in the medical and nursing world has had unforeseen consequences. Stigmatisation of patients arose in medical circles just as in the world at large, particularly in the early years when the infection was limited principally to homosexual men. AIDS has strong metaphorical associations. The diagnosis carries a fear of contamination and death, and thus quickly leads to negative moral reactions to the associated risk behaviours. People in the caring professions feared contamination, adherence to strict codes of confidentiality were thrown in doubt, and many were psychologically burdened by the care of young sick people for whom there seemed to be no hope of cure and little to offer even in the way of palliation. 'Atrocity' stories of poor treatment or frank rejection of patients quickly surfaced (Cooke, 1986). Although these were reported most commonly for doctors, nurses and other paramedical workers were not exempt. Accounts of patients left unattended, orderlies refusing to deliver meals to their bedsides, and home carers refusing to visit, quickly grew.

The theme of this chapter will be the expertise and attitudes of health professionals to AIDS as well as to people at risk of infection, their reactions to caring for people with HIV infection, and the difficulties for those who are infected with HIV themselves. Although not specifically psychiatric in nature, the attitudes and reactions of professional carers are crucial to the psychological health of sufferers. Reactions of health professionals may be emotional and inappropriate. A perception of negative reactions from professional carers can be devastating for patients who presume that health care is unprejudiced and available to all. AIDS prevention also means that doctors must be prepared to discuss personal, psychological and sexual issues with their patients where these might previously have been avoided. The emotional stress incurred by health workers in caring for patients with AIDS is considered in Chapter 10 which deals with psychological and social issues for carers, friends and families.

Britain and the USA led the world in the investigation of attitudes and knowledge of doctors, particularly of those working in primary care. The greatest problem with much of this work is the response rate of health professionals approached to take part in studies. It is dubious to generalise findings from a survey, as is so often the case, simply on the basis that there were no major differences in sociodemographic factors between responders and non-responders. These sorts of comparisons may be inadequate in determining whether the sample is self-selected or otherwise biased in terms of the attitudes or behaviours measured in the study. With this important caveat in mind, the attitudes of doctors around the world to people with HIV infection will be considered in greater detail.

Early work in the United States

One of the earliest North American surveys of the attitudes of doctors took place in 1984 in Los Angeles (Lewis et al., 1986). Primary care physicians were surveyed about their knowledge of HIV infection, screening tests and risk behaviours; their practice with patients with HIV infection; their ability to take a sexual history, and their counselling practices. Sixty-three per cent of the doctors agreed to be interviewed by telephone, the majority of whom appeared to have major gaps in their knowledge and competence, which unfortunately showed little change even after the provision of a free, continuing education programme. The same research team surveyed a further group of primary care practitioners, selected in a stratified manner from across the state of California in an attempt to generalise their findings (Lewis, Freeman & Corey, 1987). Sixty per cent were interviewed by telephone about their knowledge, attitudes and skills in the AIDS field, their views on treating gay patients and the extent of their post-graduate education on AIDS. Although reporting concern about the level of knowledge of doctors, the authors concluded that there had been at least some increase in the knowledge and competence of doctors in this area since their earlier survey. Higher levels of competence were associated with younger doctors in group practices, experience of caring for patients with

HIV infection and reporting of little discomfort in dealing with gay patients. About one-third of doctors felt uncomfortable dealing with gay patients.

Another early American survey is of interest as it was one of the few to draw inferences from the sexual orientation of the doctors themselves (Richardson et al., 1987). Doctors selected from a gay medical group were compared with doctors on a medical register in the Los Angeles area. Surprisingly few differences in knowledge and attitudes were found, although the low response rate, at 40 per cent overall, and the fact that doctors in that region of the country might be expected to be familiar with gay lifestyles could have been important factors in the results obtained. Doctors were fearful of contamination, which was the most important reason for reluctance to treat HIV patients.

In another study, which also uncovered widespread fears of infection, 263 medical and paediatric house officers affiliated with seven New York Hospitals were surveyed in 1986 about their concerns about contracting AIDS from their patients (Link et al., 1988). This study, which achieved a 98 per cent response rate, demonstrated considerable ambivalence among the doctors, with between 30 and 48 per cent reporting concern about contamination and 25 per cent reporting that they would not continue to care for AIDS patients if given a choice.

Finally, the attitudes of a further group of American doctors were explored by use of clinical case vignettes, the results of which were reported in 1987 (Kelly et al., 1987). Post residency physicians working in a major city of each of three mid-western states were selected randomly from the listing of a medical directory. The cities were chosen to be representative 'mid-range' states in terms of AIDS prevalence. Each doctor was asked to read one of four possible case vignettes and respond to a set of attitude measures eliciting their reaction to the patient described in the vignette. Physicians considered AIDs patients, in comparison to patients with leukaemia, as more responsible for their illness, more deserving of the consequences, less deserving of sympathy, more dangerous to others and more deserving of quarantine. Furthermore, they described themselves as less willing to engage in conversation with an AIDS patient, less willing to socialise or work with an AIDS patient, and more reluctant to allow their children to visit them. Despite the strikingly negative results of this survey, there were major problems in the design. As seems to be the case for most surveys of North American health workers, the study suffered from a low response rate at 32 per cent. In addition, no account was taken of the knowledge of the physicians about AIDS, the extent of their work with HIV patients, or the level of their education about AIDS. Nevertheless, it was data like these which provoked great unease in the medical profession and community alike.

Other studies carried out in the United States throughout the mid-1980s conveyed the same message. A significant number of health professionals, particularly doctors, considered themselves at risk of infection, were anxious about treating patients, held negative attitudes to homosexuality, and considered AIDS in moral terms (Wallack, 1989; Blumenfeld, Smith & Milazzo, 1987). One study is worth mentioning in greater detail as it indicated that the situational context of the contact between patient and professional was a crucial predictor of comfort with, and willingness to treat patients with HIV infection. In 1987, Dworkin, Albrecht and Cooksey (1991) conducted an anonymous questionnaire study of 536 randomly selected health care professionals made up of physicians, nurses and social workers, from one large city teaching hospital. Health care workers' emotional reactions depended very much on the type of interaction with the patient. For all three types of professional, as the invasiveness of the patient contact increased, so did the level of worry or discomfort, regardless of their overall attitudes or degree of knowledge. Low invasiveness was defined as talking with patients while high invasiveness involved inserting intravenous apparatus. Overall, nurses were most adversely affected, but they also had the greatest frequency of invasive contact with patients. This work confirms that emotional reactions by professionals to their work cannot be explained by beliefs and attitudes alone. Unfortunately, the study did not consider possible confounding factors such as length of experience with AIDS patients, attitudes towards homosexuality, and attitudes to dying patients.

Early work in Great Britain

Early in the pandemic in the UK, concern arose about the role of doctors and their competence to deal with AIDS and issues such as the psychosexual aspects of the consultation. General practitioners were widely regarded as prejudiced and incompetent in the management of patients and it is for this reason, more than for any other, that the attitudes of this particular specialty received the earliest and greatest attention. There was particular apprehension as to whether doctors understood gay 'lifestyles' (Leach & Whitehead, 1985). A practising family physician published an account of his experience of an official complaint from the mother of a young man in his practice who died of AIDS (Norell, 1986). Although the family were well aware of the young man's homosexual orientation, this had never been disclosed to the doctors in the family practice. During his final illness, he visited his doctor and the other practitioners in the practice on several occasions, but, because of their ignorance of the possibility of HIV infection, an accurate diagnosis was delayed. After the young man's death, it was claimed by the family that the doctors had been insufficiently vigilant. Although the tone of this paper, published in a leading medical journal, highlighted the frustration and concern of the doctors, their suggestion that the mother's complaint possibly stemmed from her bitterness that her son had had the misfortune to be homosexual in the first place did little to enhance the reputation of GPs with their patients.

Leading articles soon appeared thereafter in British medical journals exhorting doctors, particularly primary care physicians, to become involved both in the care of patients, and in the prevention of the spread of infection (Bucknall, 1986; Gillon, 1987*a*,*b*; Scott, 1987; King, 1987). Principal issues were knowledge and skills, confidentiality, prejudice, and refusal to treat patients. Occasionally doctors were outspoken in their wish to reserve the right to 'decline to operate on those in whom recent or continuing infection with HIV is likely, other than in life-threatening circumstances' (Guy, 1987). Professional bodies representing nurses were quicker than their counterparts for physicians to respond to the possibility of prejudicial practice by their members. In 1986, they issued guidelines for the management of AIDS in hospitals and in the community in which it was stated that any nurse who refused to treat a patient with HIV infection would be disciplined (Royal College of Nursing Working Party on AIDS, 1986). In 1987 the Royal College of General Practitioners of Great Britain set up a working party into the role of the family physician in HIV infection (Working Party of the Royal College of General Practitioners, 1988).

One of the earliest European reports on the knowledge, attitudes and behaviour of health professionals appeared in the *Lancet* in 1987. Searle surveyed over 981 hospital and community doctors of various specialties as well as senior nurses in several London health districts (Searle, 1987). Over 75 per cent of responses to a brief postal questionnaire could be analysed. It was clear from this survey that doctors were ignorant of many of the basic facts of the infection and that they were wary of undertaking invasive procedures in patients. Over three-quarters of all doctors and senior nurses were in favour of screening homosexuals, IV drug users and attenders to STD clinics, before admitting patients to hospital. Up to half considered that informed consent was not necessary before an HIV antibody test.

In 1988 and 1989 a spate of reports appeared in the UK on the work of doctors, particularly GPs, with patients with HIV infection. All surveys were based on postal surveys of doctors in the south of England, generally in London (Anderson & Mayon-White, 1988; Milne & Keen, 1988; Boyton & Scambler, 1988; King, 1989*d*; Sibbald & Freeling, 1988). Results varied as to the questions asked and the medical populations surveyed. All achieved considerably higher responses rates than most analogous studies in the USA. In three of the reports, doctors were regarded as lacking in knowledge, prejudiced against HIV patients, homosexuals and drug users, unsure about counselling patients and in some instances prepared to test for HIV antibody without the patient's prior consent (Milne & Keen, 1988; Boyton & Scambler, 1988; Sibbald & Freeling, 1988). In two of the reports, however, more encouraging outcomes were reported with doctors already active in prevention and treatment of patients (Anderson & Mayon-White, 1988; King, 1989*d*).

In a study of patients' perceptions of their GP, King (1988) interviewed 192 hospital outpatient attenders in varying stages of HIV infection. Only one-half of the sample claimed that they had informed their GP of the infection despite, in many cases, continuing to attend for medical advice. Relatively few of those patients who had told their GP of their diagnosis had received psychological support or educational advice. Doctors, however, had practically never rejected patients. Paradoxically, a majority of patients interviewed wished that their GP could be more fully informed and take a greater role in their care, particularly in terms of psychological support. Those who were reluctant to confide in the doctor were apprehensive of his or her attitude to their diagnosis, homosexuality or drug taking. Almost half of the gay men in the study would have preferred a gay doctor, perhaps reflecting their lack of confidence in the attitudes of heterosexual GPs. Similar findings were reported in data collected in the UK about one to two years later, as part of a prospective study of 263 homosexual men with HIV infection in London (Wadsworth & McCann, 1992).

Early work in other parts of the world

In Australia, 527 doctors working in a range of specialties in the state of Victoria in 1986 were surveyed by telephone about their work with HIV patients (Paine & Briggs, 1988). In general, the doctors were prepared to treat and counsel patients. Although their knowledge about the infection was patchy, particularly that of the surgeons and psychiatrists, there was little evidence of prejudiced attitudes. In keeping with other surveys around the world, the greatest difficulty was reported in counselling homosexual or bisexual men about safer sexual practices. Further work in Australia carried out in 1988 by a working party incorporating many faculties and colleges of Australian medicine led to less optimistic conclusions (Commonwealth AIDS Research Grant Committee Working Party, 1990). Of 655 general practitioners, 486 responded. Only 22 per cent, however, had treated patients with HIV infection in their practice. Although the majority regarded screening and education of patients as their role, 24 per cent did not want to maintain a therapeutic relationship with HIV patients, and 16 per cent considered it appropriate to refuse to treat such people. Lack of time was given as the commonest reason for failing to assess risk-taking behaviours routinely in their patients. Most wanted more knowledge of the illness, factors in transmission and counselling skills.

Interestingly, in Sweden, it has been reported that homosexual doctors have had a high profile and have been responsible in part for the positive changes in attitudes towards, and care of, HIV patients which have occurred in that country (Bird, 1988). However, to my knowledge, no empirical study of Swedish doctors' attitudes or behaviour has been undertaken.

Recent work world-wide

Have the attitudes and practice of doctors changed significantly in recent years The answer is a qualified 'yes'. There is now considerable evidence that GPs are caring for patients unprejudicedly, particularly in terms of day-to-day support, counselling and education (King, 1989*a*; Shapiro, 1989; Naji et al., 1989; Mansfield & Singh, 1989; Gallagher et al., 1990; Rhodes et al., 1989; Roderick, Victor & Beardow, 1990). Some reports, however, continue to indicate that doctors underestimate the degree of their patients' risk, continue to fear contamination, continue to hold negative attitudes or lack confidence in counselling (Boyd et al., 1990; Bresolin et al., 1990). A recent study from the US, designed to examine the current experiences and opinions of a national sample of family physicians with regard to AIDS, indicates little change on earlier work (Bredfeldt et al., 1991). Of 1044 doctors, 757 responded to the survey. Of these, 47 per cent had cared for an HIV-infected patient. Paradoxically, although 77 per cent of the physicians were willing to provide care to HIV-infected individuals, 63 per cent considered that physicians had a right to refuse to care for seropositive patients. Forty per cent believed that they would lose patients if it were known that they were caring for an AIDS patient in their office. Most of those doctors surveyed favoured partner notification, and would inform the sexual partner of an HIV-positive patient if the patient refused to do so.

In countries other than the USA and Britain, assessment of the work of doctors and nurses has been more patchy. Continental countries are hampered by low response rates, exemplified by a recent survey of French physicians of whom only 16 per cent responded (Pradier et al., 1991) Nevertheless, results of surveys in which satisfactory response rates are obtained demonstrate similar concerns to those already described, albeit with an increasing sensitivity and willingness to be involved. A recent Swiss study achieved a response rate of 63 per cent for a postal questionnaire of 1112 doctors in a range of specialties (Meystre-Agustoni et al., 1990). Between 40 and 70 per cent of doctors, depending on specialty, had patients with HIV infection under their care. Though the vast majority believed that they had a fundamental role to play in the prevention of HIV infection, this study revealed many persisting problems. Two-thirds admitted to some degree of difficulty in addressing the intimate sexual concerns of their patients. Almost one-half favoured public health control measures for people with HIV infection. Nine per cent believed that they ran a greater than negligible risk of contracting HIV from their patients. As to their preventive efforts, doctors tended to concentrate on homosexuals and drug users, and ignored other young, sexually active adults. Younger doctors were better informed and more prepared to act.

Regarding surveys of the needs and attitudes of patients, there is also equivocal evidence of change for the better in the relationship between patients and their doctors, although not all studies are directly comparable as they originate from different countries. The study by King (1988) of patients' attitudes towards their primary care physicians in London was replicated more recently in the cities of Munich and Berlin, Germany. Patients in Germany had higher levels of confidence in their GPs than their counterparts in Britain (Kochen et al., 1991). In a questionnaire study of 402 patients with HIV infection and AIDS, two-thirds of whom were homosexual men, it was reported that, for 91 per cent of patients, their GP was aware of the diagnosis, 81 per cent considered that their doctor had enough time for them, and 84 per cent were highly satisfied with the service provided by their GP. Nevertheless, while two-thirds would consult their GP for physical problems, only 13 per cent would do so for psychological difficulties, preferring instead to use friends or self-help groups. Although primary care physicians are well placed to provide psychological help for patients, many patients do not appear to regard such consultations as appropriate.

The learning needs of doctors

In a survey of GPs working in the neighbourhood of one of the main hospital centres for AIDS care in London, it was reported that 60 per cent wanted more education about how to deal with a wide range of aspects of HIV (Roderick et al., 1990). In this group of doctors, who potentially had easy access to a centre of considerable expertise, greatest learning needs were for estimating the probability that someone with HIV infection might develop AIDS, facts about AZT treatment, and when to refer patients to hospital. These doctors also wanted seminars on counselling and one-third would have liked actually to attend sessions in the clinic for sexually transmitted diseases.

Fortunately, efforts are under way to educate doctors about AIDS. Few, however, are evaluated in a consistent way. A recent pilot study of small-group teaching of family doctors in London is one example of what can be done (Sibbald et al., 1991). Forty-one physicians and 33 primary care nurses took part in workshops in four sites. Each workshop lasted one day and was made up of lectures, small group discussions, role play and other clinical exercises. Questionnaire evaluation at the start and finish of the day showed a significant improvement in attitudes towards prevention and management of HIV infection. Participants were more prepared to offer advice about AIDS, to negotiate safer sex and IV drug use with patients, to counsel homosexuals and drug users, to care for people with infection and their families and to introduce consistent protocols for infection control into their practices. Unfortunately, the evaluation was not controlled, no follow-up assessment after the training day was carried out, and there was no attempt to monitor actual behaviour of the workers once they were back in their practices. Nevertheless, it was an important indicator of ways in which the fears, attitudes and behaviours of health professionals might be changed.

Attitudes and behaviour of mental health professionals

Reactions by staff in the mental health specialties have also been uncertain. As is the case in other specialties, conclusions are hindered by uncertainty about response rates to surveys, the unvalidated nature of many survey questionnaires and the bias inherent to medical publication. The reality of medical journalism is that calm, unprejudiced, efficient and effective treatment in many units around the world passes unnoticed while accounts of unsatisfactory management or even open hostility to patients catches the medical headlines.

Early in the pandemic in the USA, it readily became apparent that staff of psychiatric units were apprehensive of patients with HIV infection and were ill prepared to deal with them. Polan, Hellerstein and Amchin (1985) published an account of four patients admitted to an acute psychiatric facility in Manhattan, of whom two had HIV infection and two were deluded that they were infected with the virus. Staff reactions were panicky with the emergence of open hostility and subsequent hyponchondriacal fears. Patients tended to be isolated and, although AIDS was much discussed among staff members themselves, the subject was avoided with the patients. In a similar account of an AIDS patient admitted to a psychiatric unit, Rosse (1985) reported the results of a questionnaire survey of the staff directly involved. Anxieties were related to a belief that AIDS was easily communicable, and the patient tended to be avoided by the staff. Selzer & Prince (1985) presented a similar case report of a black woman with HIV infection, consequent on IV drug use, who was admitted to a psychiatric unit with an acute psychosis. Interestingly, it was claimed that this admission highlighted the stresses already existing in the unit of racism, sexism, conflicts within and between disciplines, and the strain of working with difficult patients. Other similar reports have reached essentially similar conclusions (Cummings, Rapaport & Cummings, 1986).

Baer et al. (1987) described an approach to the psychiatric care of AIDS patients on a mental health unit specially allocated for that purpose. Their programme incorporated education of staff with the provision of forums for ventilation of concerns. This type of care which can involve extensive medical, as well as psychiatric involvement by staff, may be particularly difficult, and needs an adaptable approach by all personnel.

Reviews published some time later in the United Kingdom (Fenton, 1987) and in the USA (Binder, 1987) highlighted many of these early issues, namely refusal to admit HIV patients, fears of contamination of staff and other patients, the dilemma of treating possibly severe physical disorder, and the use of mental health legislation in patients refusing medical care. It was clear that psychiatric staff required education and training in exactly similar ways to the staff working in other specialties. Guidelines soon appeared in Britain, and in the USA, for psychiatric staff concerning confidentiality, HIV testing of psychiatrically disturbed patients and the use of mental health legislation (Catalan et al., 1989; APA, 1988*a*). Essentially, it was recommended that HIV patients should receive equivalent psychiatric care to other patients, disclosure of a patient's HIV status should be limited only to those directly involved in the care, HIV testing should be performed only with informed consent when medically indicated and not as a routine screening process, all inpatients should be considered as potentially at risk for transmitting or acquiring HIV, and that isolation or restraint of HIV patients should take place only under the most extreme circumstances, such as when patients threatened to place others at risk by their behaviour. Both sets of guidelines also emphasised the importance of staff education regarding psychiatric presentations of HIV disease as well as essentials about infectivity and routes of transmission. The guidelines produced by the American Psychiatric Association of North America have recently been revised (APA, 1992*a*,*b*), emphasising that it is inappropriate to retain patients in hospital solely for the purpose of quarantine. Despite the useful debate which has led to these documents, the possibility of HIV infection is often not considered on psychiatric units even in centres where actual prevalence is relatively high. In a recent American study of one psychiatric inpatient unit, it was demonstrated, utilising available waste bloods, that 25 (7 per cent) of 350 acutely ill patients had HIV infection, of whom ten went undetected (Sacks et al., 1992). Patients with recorded risk factors such as drug use were seldom tested. It was unclear whether HIV infection in these ten patients was of relevance to their psychiatric conditions.

It is uncertain whether staff attitudes on psychiatric units have improved in recent times. Much will depend on their experience and thus indirectly on the prevalence of HIV infection in the population served by the unit. Despite early fears of enormous demands on psychiatry by patients with HIV infection, such apprehensions have generally not been realised. Most cases are managed on medical units by liaison psychiatric doctors and nurses who frequently develop particular expertise in the field.

Attitudes of doctors and nurses toward homosexuality

Prior to the advent of AIDS, comparatively little work had been carried out into the attitudes to homosexuality of health professionals. Despite changes in attitudes of society paralleling more liberal legislation concerning male homosexual behaviour in many western countries, homosexual men and women were barely considered to have any particular need in the health services, excepting services for sexually transmitted diseases. These 'Cinderella' services were particularly sensitive to the lifestyles of homosexual people, but little empirical investigation took place. The data that are available concerning the health care of homosexual men and women before AIDS indicate that health professionals and patients alike were embarrassed to deal with issues concerning sexuality, and that patients were usually not open about their sexuality. Two studies carried out in the 1980s before AIDS, one in the USA and one in the UK, exemplify the issues.

Dardick and Grady (1980) surveyed 622 gay men and women by circulating a questionnaire in a gay news magazine in Boston, Massachusetts. The aim of the study was to explore respondents' relationships with their primary health care providers, interpreted widely to mean physician, dentist, nurse practitioner or staff member of a self-help clinic. Although only 23 per cent of questionnaires were returned, introducing a likely bias to the findings, the study is considered because it is one of the few of its kind before AIDS. Just under half of subjects had been open about their homosexuality with their primary care provider while another 11 per cent assumed that the health professional was aware of the fact. Only 7 per cent were adamant that they would not divulge the information under any circumstances. Those people whose primary care professional knew of their homosexuality were more likely to be satisfied with the care received, and to have been checked for a sexually transmitted disease. Perhaps not surprisingly, people who were open in this medical setting were also more likely to be open about their sexuality in general. Although the findings of the study were reasonably positive, over one-quarter of respondents reported having had previous experience of a health professional who was prejudiced against them, and 21 per cent considered their current health worker unsupportive. The authors recommended that health workers avoid assuming the sex of a patient's partner or assuming that, if a woman is not having sexual intercourse she must be celibate.

The second study was an anonymous survey of a stratified sample of doctors in the UK about their knowledge of, and attitudes towards, homosexuality (Bhugra & King, 1989). Again, although this study suffered from a low response rate, subgroups were matched to allow comparisons between specialties. This was the first study of its kind in which a group of homosexual doctors were included in the survey and in which the views of all the doctors were compared to a comparison group of homosexual men not in the medical profession. The data were collected in 1983, just before AIDS was generally perceived to be a problem in Britain. Although the doctors were not particularly prejudiced, psychiatrists held more liberal views than family physicians. In general, the heterosexual doctors held uninformed views of sexuality and many of them expressed a desire for more information. They believed that their medical training had left them unskilled to cope with this aspect of their patients' lives.

Since the appearance of AIDS there has been increasing concern about prejudice against homosexual people, although the amount of empirical research is surprisingly small. The attitudes of governments or research bodies towards research proposals for the study of sexuality and behaviour have not always been favourable and, in the United Kingdom, large studies with considerable public health merit have been blocked. Furthermore, reports of hostility on the part of health professionals towards homosexuals persist. As recently as 1988, gay and lesbian groups, including doctors, were calling attention to problems in the health services for homosexual people and the psychological consequences of this type of discrimination (Raymond, 1988*a*,*b*).

Although there is some evidence that attitudes to homosexual men and women have hardened since the AIDS epidemic, it has become increasingly difficult to extricate attitudes and knowledge about homosexuality from that of AIDS. A small British study of medical students demonstrated that attitudes towards AIDS patients correlated with the students' attitudes to homosexuality but not with their knowledge of AIDS (Morton & McManus, 1986). Health professionals have been forced to take account of gay lifestyles as at no time in the past. With astonishing speed, the sexuality, affections and emotions of a large minority of society became the focus for preventive efforts against AIDS and in the treatment of the disease itself. The reactions of doctors have been mixed. In services accustomed to minority groups this has not been a problem and adjustment occurred without much in the way of negative reaction (Volberding, 1980). In others, particularly those in primary care, there have undoubtedly been problems.

Several recent studies in the USA have claimed to demonstrate that health professionals are prejudiced against homosexual patients, although, in most studies, there have been design problems which throw doubt on the conclusions reached. In 1985, Douglas, Kalman and Kalman published a small report entitled *Homophobia among physicians and nurses* in which the attitudes towards homosexuality of junior doctors and nurses working in a large New York teaching hospital were measured. Only 41 per cent of physicians and 35 per cent of nurses responded to the questionnaire, although all had cared for at least one male homosexual with AIDS.

Although these health professionals were said to hold attitudes to homosexuality approximately equivalent to those of other non-medical populations among whom the questionnaire had been used previously, 31 per cent admitted that they had felt more negatively about homosexuality since the arrival of AIDS. Not surprisingly, having a gay friend, relative or colleague influenced attitudes positively towards homosexuality. It remains completely unknown whether the results could be extrapolated to the whole population of health professionals originally sampled or even whether the attitudes reported influenced their approach to patients, Nevertheless, it is unfortunately true that studies such as this can influence opinion and can alienate patients from doctors.

More reliable studies with less sensational titles have also reported on medical and nursing opinion about homosexuality as part of larger surveys of attitudes towards, and knowledge about, AIDS. Several of the studies of doctors, already referred to, have addressed this question. The principal problem appears to be a discomfort or uncertainty in dealing with sexual issues, particularly those personal to the patient (Paine & Briggs, 1988; Rhodes et al., 1989). Finally, Ross and Hunter have recently published a fear of AIDS schedule in which they report that health professionals' fear of contamination through blood or illness rather than any fear of homosexuals or bisexuals leads to avoidance of AIDS patients (Ross & Hunter, 1991). However, as it was uncertain how their small, mainly female, sample of health professionals was chosen, their conclusions must remain tentative.

Thus, despite occasional reports (Milne & Keen, 1988), usually based on attitude questionnaires of unestablished validity, there is little evidence from in-depth studies of pervasive antagonism towards homosexuals (King, 1989*a*), although it is clear that patients are apprehensive about the likelihood of such attitudes (King, 1988; Mansfield & Singh, 1989).

Health professionals and drug users

Similar work has been conducted into the work of health professionals with drug users. Here the picture is clearer, albeit depressing. In general, it can be said that attitudes of doctors, nurses and paramedics, not directly involved in services for drug users, are almost universally hostile. Clearly, such attitudes will have major ramifications for the prevention and treatment of AIDS.

Although it is frequently asserted that doctors, particularly family physicians, should be more prepared to deal with drug users (Richards,

1988; Dole, 1989), most recent surveys continue to indicate their profound unpopularity with doctors. In 1985, Glanz surveyed a random sample of general practitioners in England and Wales about their attitudes towards, and the extent of their contact with, opiate users (Glanz, 1986*a*,*b*; Glanz & Taylor, 1986). One in five of the doctors surveyed had been consulted by an opiate user in the preceding four weeks; two-thirds of the users had consulted the doctor for assistance with withdrawal or rehabilitation. Although about one-third of the 845 doctors who responded to the survey were prescribing opiates, it was unclear to what extent this took place independently of the specialist drug services. Doctors usually preferred to direct patients to other services than deal with the drug problem themselves. The doctors regarded opiate users as difficult to manage, beyond their competence to treat, and less acceptable than other patients. Two-thirds regarded opiate dependence as symptomatic of an underlying personality disorder. On a more optimistic note, younger family physicians were more ready to be involved, and were more confident in their ability to deal with users. Many more doctors were prepared to take on drug users, given better backing by specialist drug services.

Since this study was carried out, drug services in Britain have continued to respond to the AIDS crisis with the development of community drug teams of counsellors and drug specialists who liaise more directly with doctors. Nevertheless, the little data that is available indicate that drug users remain unpopular with doctors. Investigation of the burden of care for doctors have been conflicting. Some authors have claimed that heroin users consult their family doctors for reasons similar to those of other patients, and only a few make heavy demands (Neville et al., 1988), while others have reported sharp increases in consultation rates for drug users over the mid- to late 1980s (Roberts, Skidmore & Robertson, 1989). It is likely that GPs' involvement with drug users will escalate as community drug services increasingly maintain users on oral opiates outside of traditional clinic settings and seek prescriptions from the patient's doctor to do so. Thus, the role of the primary care physician will become increasingly important, and there is a need for continuing education to change attitudes and good lines of communication with specialist staff (Brettle, 1987).

Insufficient investigation has been conducted into the views and perceived needs for health care of the drug users themselves, who are simply regarded by doctors, at least, as single minded in their pursuit of drugs (see Chapter 7). In recent years occasional surveys of the views of drug users have been published but usually in the context of AIDS services and HIV testing

(Curtis et al., 1989). More detailed examination of their physical and psychological needs will assist planning of services, education of doctors and the understanding of drug dependence.

Health professionals with HIV infection

A continuing controversy besets the ability of doctors and nurses who are HIV positive to continue to work. Just as the risk posed to health workers by their patients is extremely low, if the necessary precautions are adopted (Friedland et al., 1986; McEvoy et al., 1987), risk to patients from seropositive doctors is correspondingly tiny. Nevertheless, in an infection where new information is constantly emerging, experts have been forced to revise their opinion on many points, a fact which undermines credibility in this sensitive area (Gerbert et al., 1988). Although a trivial risk, it is, nevertheless, a risk of a very serious infection and requires further surveillance (Bird et al., 1991).

There is considerable discussion both in the United States and in Europe, concerning the risk posed by infected health care professionals in the wake of the case of a dentist who is believed to have passed the virus on to five of his patients before his own death from AIDS. In the United Kingdom, newspapers have published the identity of doctors who have died of AIDS (Black, 1987) and in some cases, have only been prevented from identifying doctors with HIV infection publicly by High Court injunctions (Dyer, 1987). Official recommendations have, however, been somewhat inconsistent. As early as 1987, the United States Center for Disease Control issued a statement to the effect that it needed to be determined on an individual basis whether HIV infected health care workers should continue to work or whether their duties should be altered. At the same time, the British Medical Association was advising doctors with HIV infection not to perform invasive procedures (Adler, 1987). The Department of Health in the UK has issued guidelines for infected health professionals which make their responsibilities more explicit, while continuing to emphasise the lack of evidence that patients are placed at any significant risk (Department of Health, 1991).

In July 1991, the United States Senate mandated draconian measures involving ten-year prison sentences and fines of $10 000 for health care workers who are aware that they are seropositive but who do not inform patients upon whom they perform invasive procedures. The Senate went even further, however, in requiring all doctors and dentists performing 'high risk' operations to be tested for HIV infection (Morris, 1991). At the annual meeting of the American Medical Association in June 1991, the former American Vice-President, Dan Quayle, supported compulsory HIV testing for doctors and their patients. Despite these ill-informed panic statements, we must continue to be reminded that coercive testing can only lead to an unprecedented invasion of privacy, loss of confidentiality and possible discrimination (Morris, 1991). Furthermore, it is currently unwarranted; only one health care professional, the dentist already referred to, has been known to pass on infection to his patients.

The issue for seropositive health workers is more complicated, however, than simply the risk of passing on the infection. They are subject to the same psychological stresses as experienced by other people with HIV, and the possibility of cognitive impairment and loss of judgement is perceived as a possible threat to their professional competence. In addition, doctors who have contracted AIDS through their work have occasionally become stigmatised and the source of infection disputed. This uncertainty, together with the fear of being publicly exposed, places enormous strain on those doctors, nurses and other health workers who happen to be seropositive.

To my knowledge, there has been no empirical study of health professionals who are infected with HIV, not least because of the difficulties of enlistment and confidentiality. Anecodotal evidence would suggest that, although many people with HIV infection seek to work with patients, either in a voluntary capacity or in the health services, insufficient study has been made of their particular difficulties. It takes little imagination to realise that serious stress might occur more quickly and severely in such people who are confronted daily with the results of an infection that they themselves harbour. Similar notions might apply to homosexual men or drug users who are involved in the caring professions dealing with AIDS. In their study of the psychological effects, for physicians, of treating patients with AIDS, Horstman and McKusick (1986) reported that gay doctors were more stressed but the authors did not, or could not, take account of the seropositivity of the physicians. Clearly, such studies are more difficult to undertake, but the information is of potential importance, as this group of health workers might be expected to be more vulnerable and thus in need of greater support.

Conclusions

What level of consensus can be drawn from this broad field? We must continue to educate professionals in all health fields and to monitor their attitudes and behaviour. Monitoring has tended to be neglected in recent years. Doctors need to feel competent in enquiring about, and advising on, sexual matters, to improve their knowledge about drug use and to incorporate more counselling into their work. A minispecialty among general practitioners who are expert in the field of AIDS is probably inevitable. Rather than expect all doctors to be expert, we might do better to concentrate on ensuring that all doctors have competence in the knowledge and skills necessary for prevention of HIV infection. We need to be vigilant against discrimination in our services, be it against patients or professionals. It is clear that fears of contamination persist at some level even among some of our most experienced health workers and it may be unrealistic to expect that it can be removed altogether. A certain level of alertness is important to ensure that health professionals adopt appropriate safe procedures. Clearer guidelines are required for infected health professionals as are wider public education efforts to stem inappropriate concern about transmission from professional to patient.

CHAPTER TEN

CONSEQUENCES FOR PROFESSIONALS, INFORMAL CARERS, FRIENDS, AND FAMILIES

No illness concerns only the sufferer, there are emotional, social and economic repercussions for the *entourage*. As in any other potentially life-threatening condition, people infected with HIV may place considerable psychological and social demands on those who care for them as well as on those with whom they have close social ties. Although often coping with the challenge, those closest to the patient encounter particular needs of their own. In the early part of this chapter, I will return to the theme of the health professional, but, in this instance, to consider the burden that providing care imposes on the provider. This will be followed by an appraisal of the issues for informal carers, families and friends. Finally, bereavement issues which are specific to HIV will be considered.

Stress in health professionals working with people with HIV

AIDS, in common with other serious diseases, may cause marked distress not only in patients and their immediate family and friends but also in their professional care-givers. Doctors and nurses may react with fearful apprehension, or become emotionally overwhelmed by the complexity of treatment and inevitable outcome of the disorder. Not only are young people dying in their care, but they are also suffering a stigmatised disorder which introduces new strains into the traditional relationship between staff and patients and their families, friends and partners. Health workers may sometimes be placed under enormous pressure to maintain divided confidentialities and loyalties and they may be the first to be blamed when these go awry. In similar fashion, they may readily become the targets of displaced grief. The result of such pressures for many staff may be psychological distress leading to over-identification with patients or neglect of their normal care, evasion of emotional issues, avoidance of dying patients or hypochondriacal fears of infection. This may lead on to prolonged sick leave or resignation from the service. The stress for health professionals, who are themselves infected with HIV, is likely to be even more severe. However, the burden which HIV care imposes on health professionals can only be put in the context of what is already known about their psychological health, apart from AIDS. Health professionals appear to be a stressed group.

Stress in health professionals

There is nothing particularly new about the concept of stress reactions in the work-place. There has been extensive study of the psychological reactions of health care workers, who have traditionally been regarded as a vulnerable group because of the nature of their work. Most examination of this issue has been conducted on doctors, somewhat less on nurses. Concern about the psychological health of doctors has led to several editorials in leading British medical journals in recent years (Rawnsley, 1986; Mayou, 1987; Lask, 1987; Pilowsky & O'Sullivan, 1989). Rates of suicide for doctors are approximately two to three times that of populations of comparable social class (Anon., 1964; Richings, Khara & McDowell, 1986; Rose & Rosow, 1973), although no particular specialty predominates (Rose & Rosow, 1973). Substance abuse may be up to 30 times more common among doctors than in the general population (Rucinski & Cybulska, 1985) with estimates that up to 1 per cent of all American physicians may be dependent on drugs (Waring, 1974). Rates for admission for alcoholism among doctors in the UK exceed those of people of similar social class (Murray, 1976), and outcome in terms of social and occupational functioning is poor. Medical students, never particularly renowned for their temperance, continue to drink at levels that may place them at risk for later addiction (Collier & Beales, 1989). In a longitudinal study spanning 30 years of adult life, Vaillant, Sobowale & McArthur (1972) reported that doctors had poorer marriages, were more likely to abuse alcohol and use sedatives, tranquillisers or stimulants than those in other professions. They were also more likely to have sought psychotherapy. There have been claims that psychological disorder among doctors is often related to early life problems and adjustment *prior* to professional training (Vaillant et al., 1972; Arana, 1982) and some have gone so far as to make the controversial suggestion of screening out vulnerable personalities at application to medical school (a'Brook, 1967). Levels of emotional distress among junior doctors are known to be high, and have been related to the particular demands of this part of medical training (Firth-Cozens, 1987). However, despite an extensive literature, we remain unsure of the exact levels of emotional distress among doctors who are beyond their junior years. Reported prevalence of emotional distress, variously defined, ranges between 0.5 and 46 per cent reflecting the difficulties inherent to this type of research. Doctors may be reluctant to admit to problems (particularly substance abuse), and studies have been hampered by methodological problems (Waring, 1974).

Study of the problems for nurses before the advent of AIDS is less common and concentrates more closely on work-related stress, rather than on the wider issues of mental health. Nevertheless, many of the findings for doctors are echoed in this group. For example, Gary-Toft and Anderson (1981) studied stress in 122 nurses from hospice, and a range of other medical and surgical, settings. Overwork, managing dying patients and an inability to meet the emotional demands of patients were the principal concerns of these nurses. Interestingly, hospice nurses seemed to be best adapted. In a large study of 1800 intensive care nurses, principal stresses highlighted were difficulties with management, interpersonal relationships and patient care (Bailey, Stefen & Grout, 1980).

Burnout

The term 'burnout' arose in the 1970s to describe the process of demoralisation and decompensation that may occur under severe and chronic stress at work. More recently, it has been limited to mean a syndrome of emotional exhaustion and cynicism which occurs in people who work with people (Maslach & Jackson, 1981). The syndrome is classically one of chronic frustration in a work situation leading to lowered morale, neglect of normal responsibilities and a flattened, disinterested response to further stress. Burned out individuals have little emotion left to give to either their patients or their family and friends. Unfortunately, the introduction of this term, which begs the question of what was burning in the first place, has added little to the understanding of reactions to work stress.

What is known about the effects on health professionals of working with patients with AIDS? Despite much anecdotal reporting, until recently, there has been suprisingly little systematic attempt to determine the psychological adjustment of medical and paramedical staff working with AIDS patients. Even in the work reported, which has been primarily descriptive in nature, methodological problems prevent ready acceptance of the results. Furthermore, we have little understanding of the nature of the stressors, let alone their effects. Research into 'shop floor' issues, such as the hour-to-hour burden of work expected of staff, rôle conflicts and the command hierachy, might be as profitable as detailed examination of the symptoms of burnout, if we are to alter the fundamental causes.

The interpretation of findings based on questionnaires which purport to measure stressful issues for staff are hampered by problems of faulty recall and doubtful validity. Potentially more interesting, qualitative study of the reports of individuals or groups of carers encounter difficulties of analysis and small sample sizes. In either qualitative or quantative studies, the validity of self-report is also limited by the possibility that responders may wish to avoid admitting distress for fear of being considered weak or vulnerable, or they may wish to exaggerate the stress involved for other reasons.

Perhaps the most well-known, quantitative work in this field is that by Maslach & Jackson (1981), who derived a self-report questionnaire designed to measure frequency and intensity of perceived attitudes and emotions towards work-related stressors. Twenty-two items were generated by factor analysis from a larger pool collected to measure emotional exhaustion, depersonalisation and personal accomplishment. This latter factor is important in that it balances the negative factors by incorporating the possibility of positive gain from work. The questionnaire was constructed using a total sample of 1025 people from the helping professions interpreted widely to include health and social service workers, the police and teachers. It was reported that questionnaire scores were closely correlated with behavioural ratings of subjects made by other people who knew them well, job characteristics which might lead to stress and personal habits and feelings about work satisfaction assessed using other self-reports. An attempt was also made to discriminate burnout from ordinary job dissatisfaction not related to chronic stress.

Thus this inventory was carefully constructed along conventional lines and has since been applied in the AIDS field. It has to be said, however, that, as in all such work in the psychological or social domain the concept of burnout used in the first place must be, at least in part, a product of the authors' own views on work-related stress. The pool of questions were derived from assessments of the attitudes and feelings which 'characterise the burned out worker' and thus, of necessity, the resulting questionnaire incorporates their views of what comprises such a syndrome in the first place. Direct measurement of stress by physiological recording of heart rate and ectopic beats, or skin conductance are possible and have been applied in other professions (Douglas et al., 1988). They remain, nevertheless, physiological recordings whose applicability to the concept of chronic emotional overload or burnout are theoretical at best.

Unfortunately, much of the research on stress in professionals working with AIDS has omitted to include any comparison with other groups working in other specialties, a problem which renders the data much less useful. A further important issue which has received little attention, at least in the empirical literature, is the concept of salience of the health issue. It is rarely considered why people enter the health field, in general, and AIDS care, in particular. It would seem, at least in the voluntary sector, that people are drawn to work in a specific field because they identify personally with the needs of patients who suffer from that disorder. This is nowhere more evident than in AIDS care where many homosexual men and women, drug users and HIV-infected individuals have taken a leading role in social and health care. The impact of caring for dying patients is likely to be different on people who identify with the epidemic, or feel personally under threat from it. A final point, which is seldom addressed, is that of vulnerable personalities. Whether a number of health care workers are also personally vulnerable to stress for other reasons, and are thus drawn to the health field as a vicarious way of gaining help, is much more difficult to study and can be a threatening issue to address. These points will be returned to in the discussion of research which follows.

The evidence

One of the earliest reports of the effect of AIDS on health staff came from the USA (Horstman & McKusick, 1986). One hundred and fifty San Francisco Bay Area physicians from a range of specialties who treated patients with HIV disease were posted a questionnaire of whom 82 (55 per cent) responded. Forty were also interviewed. Sixty-three percent were homosexual men and women. Although it was unclear how the sample was selected for the study, these doctors were heavily involved with AIDS care. On average, they had been working with HIV patients for three years and spent over 40 per cent of their week in contact with such patients. Over half reported more stress, and over 40 per cent more fear of death and anxiety, since working with AIDS. Although length of experience in AIDS care was not related to distress, amount of contact with patients was directly correlated with psychological distress. It seems that concentrated exposure to patients, rather than years of exposure, is the critical factor in emotional reactions to the work. Periods away from patients are clearly an important protective factor against stress in health professionals in this field. Those patients whom doctors found most difficult to manage were hypochondriacal men who sought constant reassurance. When dealing with very sick people, repeated requests for reassurance about minor symptoms from others made the doctors very impatient. Despite these findings, over 40 per cent reported that involvement in AIDS care had given them greater intellectual and career satisfaction. Homosexual physicians were more stressed than their heterosexual counterparts. Principal methods of coping with stress were talking to friends, partners or family members. Use of medication or alcohol was much less likely. Although about half relied on colleagues for support, few expressed a desire for support groups of doctors meeting to discuss work-related stress.

Although there have been subsequent studies of the psychological consequences of caring for patients with HIV infection, some have applied uncertain methods while others have focused on very small numbers of staff. In a survey of mainly nurses and paramedical staff in two major teaching hospitals in Australia, Ross & Seeger (1988) reported that, although up to 40 per cent of staff experienced significant distress in dealing with AIDS related issues, over half found that the intellectual stimulation deriving from their work served as a compensation. Sources of greatest difficulty for staff were the young age of patients, neurological aspects of the infection such as dementia, and management of dying patients. In addition, one in five staff reported persistent fears about acquiring infection despite a median time of working with AIDS patients of 18 months and a median number of AIDS-related patients of 40. Clearly, experience with patients does little to reduce fear of contamination in a significant proportion of staff and may be a chronic source of stress. Most common means of coping with stress were sharing experiences with colleagues, not discussing the problems at home, and maintaining active interests outside work. The authors suggested that the provision of peer support groups might prevent distress in staff most effectively. Two major uncertainties preclude ready acceptance of the findings of this study. No information was provided on the response rate to the survey which was anonymous, or on whether the sample was representative of all health professionals dealing with AIDS patients in the two hospitals surveyed.

In a small study which is of interest because it included a comparison between an AIDS patient and a matched patient without AIDS, Treiber, Shaw and Malcolm (1987) assessed the psychological impact on eight nurses and four physicians involved in the patients' care. The AIDS patient was perceived as being more difficult, demanding and resistive, and more anxiety provoking. Although the idea behind the study was a useful one, limiting the comparison to two particular patients made it impossible to differentiate individual personality factors from general differences due to the AIDS diagnosis.

In a small, but carefully controlled investigation of work-related stress in nurses, Bennett, Michie and Kippax (1991) compared registered nurses working with AIDS with those working in an oncology service in two large Sydney hospitals. A 95 per cent response rate was obtained, resulting in 32 nurses in AIDS and 32 nurses in oncology. Subjects completed a questionnaire concerning emotional exhaustion, depersonalisation and personal accomplishment in relation to their work. A complicated statistical analysis revealed that, although subjects working in the AIDS field did not suffer emotional exhaustion as often as in the oncology service, when it occurred, the emotional exhaustion was more intense. There were important hospital differences which implied better staff–patient ratios, opportunities for career advancement or management of stress in one than the other. However, work-related stress or burnout, the term used by the authors, was not related to the experience of the nurse but rather to their age and the amount of time spent in the unit. The older the nurse, and the less time working in the unit, the less the burnout. Although no sex differences in prevalence of stress were found, only 3 of the 32 oncology nurses were male compared with 18 of the 32 AIDS nurses.

Well-conducted, qualitative study of the reactions of medical professionals to AIDS care is less common. One exception is a small study in the USA which used careful selection criteria and methods of analysis. Thirty primary care physicians practising in six small, north-eastern cities of the USA were interviewed on the basis of having a stipulated minimum involvement in the care of patients with HIV infection. Each doctor was interviewed in depth about his or her emotional responses to death and dying in AIDS care and fears of contagion (Epstein et al., 1993). Interviews were recorded and transcribed before analysis by narrative techniques. All transcripts were collapsed into reliably identifiable themes which were subjected to more detailed analysis. Although this study suffered design problems related to the selection and response rates of the doctors taking part, and a modification of the interview format half-way through the data collection, it is of interest because it throws a particularly vivid light on the practical and emotional difficulties encountered by physicians who care for people with AIDS. Most of the doctors admitted to feelings of emotional distress, bereavement and helplessness, but only two expressed fears of burnout. Confirming the quantitative reports already discussed above, many of the doctors mentioned the positive aspects of caring for patients with AIDS, and believed that it was a special privilege to share in a patient's process of dying. Fear of contagion was common among these 30 primary care physicians, despite a reasonably accurate perception of their actual risk. Although such fears sometimes led to over-attention to infection control measures, or erratic use of precautions, they did not lead to avoidance of care for patients.

Intervention for health care workers

It is apparent that health professionals suffer emotional strain from treating young patients with terminal diseases, but it is much less apparent what can be done about it. Although Ross & Seeger (1988) proposed the establishment of peer support groups, this was not regarded as a popular option by the doctors in Horstman and McKusick's (1986) study who sought their own support from partners and friends. There are considerable problems in sustaining interdisciplinary support groups in a busy clinical environment, and staff may be reluctant to reveal their distress or vulnerability to each other. Rivalries and hierachical issues may make it difficult for senior staff to support the juniors. Similar stresses exist in other services for terminally ill patients where these issues have long been debated (Parkes, 1986). Mental health professionals may have a role to play in providing staff support on an individual or group basis but it is helpful if they are not active members of the service and work closely with other carers with special skills relevant to the task (Parkes, 1986). Although staff support groups may be a format wherein stress reduction is possible, other suggestions have included widening the range of services that accept AIDS patients in order that many more physicians and hospitals become involved (Volberding, 1989). In so doing, the burden may be shared, and experience of the condition generalised to the wider medical and nursing community. As proposed by Horstman and McKusick (1986) and Bennett et al. (1991), reducing the intensity of work in AIDS, by the taking of frequent short breaks, might go furthest in reducing stress. However, interventions will also need to deal with issues such as identification and close relationships with patients. Perhaps older, more experienced staff need to be used in AIDS units.

Stress in informal carers

Much of the treatment of patients with HIV disease takes place in the community, and relies on the availability of people close to the patient to do most of the caring. Until recently, few studies had undertaken an examination of the care provided by informal carers of patients with AIDS and the emotional and social cost they bear. McCann and Wadsworth (1992), as part of a larger study of the psychological and social consequences for homosexual men with HIV infection, contacted informal carers nominated by the men. Carers were those people regarded by the men in the study as providing them with help or care on an informal basis. Of the 265 individuals involved in the larger study, 55 per cent named at least one such carer, of whom 71 per cent were interviewed. The most common carers identified were close friends or partners. Twenty-eight per cent had health problems which often affected their ability to care. One in ten carers were HIV seropositive themselves. Over half reported that they took on most of the care of the index patient. An enormous range of practical and emotional support was provided by the carers who were sometimes under considerable strain themselves, particularly if also suffering from HIV-related problems. Carers felt least supported emotionally and often suffered social problems, particularly maintaining their own employment. The presence of an informal carer was paradoxically associated with a greater likelihood of hospital admission for the patient, perhaps as a result of early recognition of problems, more effective mobilisation of resources, or because of an acknowledgement by clinical teams of the strain imposed on the carer.

If community care is to continue to expand, specific help for carers will be required, not only for those assisting patients with HIV disease but also for all those people with chronic disorders cared for outside of hospital. In Britain, the King Edward's Hospital Fund, an organisation supporting research, audit and discussion in the health field, has published guidelines for supporting informal carers. These include recognition of their contribution and their needs, together with the provision of respite care, practical help, emotional support and a specific income which does not preclude the carer from also sustaining outside employment (King's Fund, 1989).

Stress in families

In recent times, the concept of the family has undergone considerable revision. More people live in non-traditional settings, and AIDS has accelerated this change with its impact upon kinship, housing and child custody. The structure of families range in form from couples in close, childless relationships through extended networks which include third-degree relatives. The family of an individual can be considered to be the family of origin, the spouse or partner and related offspring, together with their children. Non-coupled individuals may consider their close friends as family support. An all-encompassing definition is therefore probably not possible. Perhaps the only meaningful use of the term will include those people with whom a person has the closest emotional, social and economic bonds. For example, the family in contemporary North American society has recently been defined as a group of individuals who, by birth, adoption, marriage, or declared commitment, share deep personal connections through which they receive, and are obligated to provide, support of various kinds (Levine, 1990).

Family reactions to HIV infection vary with the nature of the transmission. Issues within families where the affected person has acquired the infection through transfusion of blood products will differ from those where they are homosexual, or a drug user, or where the infection is acquired heterosexually. All have distinct consequences which are patterned on the structure of the family that exists. It is not uncommon for gay men to be more distant from their families, both geographically and emotionally, than their heterosexual counterparts because of the difficulties many parents and siblings encounter in coming to terms with the sexual orientation of their son or brother. On occasions, parents learn of the sexual orientation of their son at the same time as the news that he has HIV infection, or is dying of AIDS. The stress for families caught in this predicament can be very severe, and subsequently interrupt the grieving process. This theme, which has formed the content of several recent cinematic films of varying quality, will be returned to in the section on bereavement which follows.

The economic consequences for the family may be very damaging in one context, particularly in developing countries, while, in others, money may be made available through bequests which, in unexpected ways may assist families previously in difficulties. In countries with little or no welfare system, when children are not accepted into the extended family network, they may become homeless and add to the already growing numbers of street children who are so vulnerable to physical and mental exploitation with consequent psychological problems and substance abuse (Gibb, Duggan & Lewin, 1991). Older members of extended families, such as grandparents, may be called upon to support their surviving grandchildren while still grieving the loss of their children and facing increasing economic hardship. There may be particular problems for the well siblings of affected children. Parents may shield the knowledge from them, as they watch their brother or sister inexplicably grow weaker. Children who are aware of the basis of the illness in their brother or sister may realise that they are also losing one or both parents, and may fear for their own health. Behavioural and emotional disturbance in the well sibling is possible, and has already been shown to occur in families where children suffer from other chronic medical complaints. The degree of disturbance, however, seems to depend on the level of overall support which is provided to the family from professional and other sources. This topic was returned to in Chapter 8 which deals with the particular needs of affected children.

Very little research has been targeted specifically at the families of people with HIV infection or AIDS, possibly for all the difficulties of definition and setting just described. Much more information is needed on the crucial components of support, patterns of caring and stigma within families affected by AIDS across differing cultural contexts. For example, the implications for the psychological and physical health of parents when the infection is first detected in a baby or infant, may be very different from those where it is found in a grown son. The demand for more research on families and AIDS is reflected in the theme of the 1992 International Conference on AIDS in Amsterdam which, for the first time, included the needs and difficulties of families.

Bereavement

Mourning involves emotional, physical and spiritual reactions which may lead people to feel abandoned, confused, depressed and sometimes suicidal. It is a time when there may be emotions of relief that the dying process is over, mingled with evocative memories, regret, loneliness and great sadness. The process occurs in stages in which the alarm incurred by the initial shock is followed by searching for the deceased, guilt and anger, leading to eventual acceptance and resolution with the development of a new identity (Parkes, 1972).

HIV infection affects young people in a generation which is not accustomed to early death. Death may lead to an increased fear of susceptibility to AIDS which was suspended during the time when the dying person required extensive support. Survivors may feel stigmatised merely by association with death (Shearer & McKusick, 1986). Nor does death release families and loved ones from the stigma and prejudice of the disease (King, 1989*c*). Deception may occur about the cause of death within families, and may lead to intolerable strain at funerals, and in the months that follow. Those people closest to the deceased may be unable to share the true nature of the death for fear of family stigma or rejection. In attempting to hide the exact cause of death from relatives, family members may experience a secretive and protracted grief. Thus, parents may suffer not only the strain of loss but also the consequences of partial disclosure to those in their family who could help them most (Shearer & McKusick, 1986). Where the cause of death is known, lovers of patients who have died may be ignored by families who reject the nature of their relationship if it was homosexual, or disapprove of it if it was heterosexual.

Homosexuality and bereavement

Gay partners who have lived with the deceased for decades may be excluded from any real sharing in the grief or, more materially, in the estate. Individuals in same sex partnerships are less likely to make valid wills and may lose shared homes and effects when one partner dies (Cave, 1983). If the family does not accept their son's relationship or the rights of his chosen partner, conflict is inevitable. In most Western countries, there is little in the way of legal redress for bereaved partners who might find themselves in such a predicament.

Although homosexual men often receive support from the gay community (Hart et al., 1990), they may be required to conceal the extent of their grief from others in their social network who are unaware of the true nature of their relationship with the deceased. The young heterosexual man who loses a wife will receive appropriate understanding from acquaintances and work colleagues and will be allowed a period of reduced responsibility within which to resolve his grief. The homosexual man will usually have to hide his loss and, even if frank about it, is likely to receive less sympathy on the implicit assumption that homosexual relationships are less emotionally and socially valid than their heterosexual counterparts.

Despite little rational foundation to the religious condemnation of either homosexuality or AIDS (Murphy, 1988), the church has long been opposed to the recognition or acceptance of gay lifestyles, and thus it is not surprising that some ministers of religion have negative views of homosexual relationships and may avoid mentioning anything of real value about the deceased at funerals or, even worse, show their embarrassment or hostility towards partners (Lack, 1990). The recent, well-publicised hostility towards homosexual clergy in the Church of England in the United Kingdom gives all the wrong signals in efforts to ameliorate society's reaction against AIDS and homosexuality.

Gay bereavement was seldom considered as a distinct phenomenon until the advent of AIDS. Although occasional reports had considered the issue in both homosexual men and women they were mainly descriptive in content (Siegal & Hoefer, 1981). Even since the appearance of AIDS, many reports have been impressionistic (Shilts, 1987). However, the bereavement that has afflicted gay communities, particularly in North America, has recently been the subject of intense enquiry, either in its own right or as a possible co-factor in disease progression or in psychological decompensation. In a detailed North American study of mainly white, homosexual men it was reported that men bereaved of a lover or close friend with AIDS, experienced symptoms of a post-traumatic stress response with intrusive thoughts and emotions about AIDS (Martin, 1988). Seven hundred and forty-five gay men recruited through a variety of sources in New York City were interviewed in the mid-1980s to determine links between bereavement and psychological distress. None of the men had a diagnosis of AIDS and only 50 knew of their antibody status at interview, 16 of whom were antibody seropositive. Twenty-seven per cent of this sample had experienced bereavement, to mean the loss of a lover or close friend with AIDS, of whom one-third had suffered multiple losses. Bereaved men were vulnerable to demoralisation and sleep problems. They were more likely to have used sedatives and consulted psychological services primarily for AIDS concerns. These findings remained significant after controlling for effects of their own compromised health status and appraised threat of AIDS.

In another, similar study conducted in 1985, 180 homosexual men who had lost a lover or close friend to AIDS during the first five years of the epidemic were interviewed (Lennon, Martin & Dean, 1990). Reaction to the bereavement was assessed using a 12-item scale developed for the study, while availability and adequacy of practical and emotional support were assessed with reference to the tasks of caretaking and emotional pain experienced during the lover's or close friend's illness with AIDS. Gay men, who lost a lover or close friend to AIDS, experienced symptoms of grief similar to those reported in studies of bereaved spouses and parents. More intense grief reactions occurred among those who had taken care of their lover or close friend during his illness. Perceived adequacy of practical and emotional support, rather than simply its availability, was strongly related to the level of grief. Men who had received inadequate help with caretaking responsibilities experienced more intense symptoms of grief subsequent to the death compared to those who reported receiving adequate caretaking support. Similarly, those men who reported receiving insufficient emotional support for the pain they experienced during the course of the illness suffered more intense symptoms of grief than those who considered that they had received adequate support.

Mental health professionals need to be aware of issues specific to gay bereavement. To do so, they must have some understanding and acceptance of homosexual ways of life (Berger, 1990). Perhaps as crucial in the process is that homosexual men and women who mourn a partner need to begin to regard themselves as worthy of the same consideration and support as heterosexuals in similar circumstances. Too often, even within the gay community, there is an internalised, implicit devaluation of the depth and significance of homosexual partnerships.

Grief and the death certificate

Death certification in many countries, including the United Kingdom, is an important mechanism by which actual cause of death may be released to others, usually for the purposes of public health statistics. However, death certificates containing the cause of death may have to be presented by family members or partners to administrators, employers and insurance companies, with consequent loss of confidentiality for the patient and embarrassment and distress for his or her relatives (King, 1989*c*). Although many doctors in the United Kingdom intentionally obscure the issue by supplying a more innocuous diagnosis on the certificate such as pneumonia, while indicating in another section of the form that further information will be available, this, albeit humane action, side-steps the issue of confidentiality after death, and leaves the possibility open for other doctors or coroners to be less understanding. All people have a right to privacy, and there is no valid reason why this should be denied them after death. Failure to pay attention to the administrative aspects of death can only complicate bereavement and the process of grief.

Conclusions

It is inevitable that those closely involved in the care of people dying with AIDS will be affected profoundly by the process. Although often not acknowledged, doctors and nurses are frequently ill prepared to face issues of death and dying in patients suffering from any serious illness. In AIDS, patients may be of similar age and social profile to their carers and the prognosis of the infection is ultimately gloomy. The term burnout has been adopted to describe the decompensation of professional carers in the face of chronic work pressures but has done little to further our understanding of the issues. Staff who may be particularly vulnerable for personal reasons, or because they are also HIV seropositive may need particular support and counselling. Although peer support may be useful in certain situations, adequate time away from intensive care of patients may do most to prevent excessive strain. It is more difficult to prepare professionals who are in training. Although teaching medical students or student nurses about the issues of death and dying is necessary and important, many of the ethical and philosophical difficulties cannot be fully understood until trainees begin work in the field, and until they have resolved their personal feelings about the issues.

Families, partners, and informal carers face even greater difficulties in that they frequently receive little training or support, are often already closely emotionally involved with the patient and may be ill themselves. Little is known about the role of the family in the care of patients with HIV infection, and this is a subject which needs urgent consideration, particularly in developing countries where an increasing burden of child care may be thrown back on older generations while the family's livelihood is progressively reduced. Bereavement in AIDS is affected by the issues of prejudice which bedevil all aspects of the disorder. Multiple bereavements are affecting gay populations in Western countries, and are devasating whole sections of the population in some African countries. These issues will have profound effects on mental health services which are associated with AIDS care.

CHAPTER ELEVEN

STRESS, PSYCHOLOGICAL DISORDER AND THE IMMUNE SYSTEM

Psychological factors have long been implicated in the function of the immune system and interest in this field has increased markedly with the appearance of AIDS. There is a common belief among patients with HIV infection that positive mental attitudes, or a fighting spirit, may have direct beneficial effects on their immune system and may delay or even prevent the onset of HIV disease. Psychological or social adversity may be a co-factor for the progression of HIV infection. This is an important area of psychosomatic research of which all mental health professionals working in the AIDS field should be aware. Much of the evidence, however, is conflicting, and derives from poorly conducted, or uncontrolled studies. Any investigation of the association between emotional stress and immune function must control for age and physical status of participants, baseline levels of ambient stress, the nature, inherent meaning and duration of the stressor, and circadian or seasonal fluctuations in immunological functioning. Studies are subject to the confounding influences on immune function of alcohol and drug use, previous infections and current treatments. The time lag between a stressor and its possible effects, and the role of homeostatic mechanisms in correcting imbalances caused by stress, are unknown. Stress itself is difficult to define or measure. With these introductory cautions in mind, this chapter will focus on the evidence for links between emotional and immune function and, most particularly, how this might influence progression in HIV infection.

The nature of stress

Like many human experiences, stress is easily recognised but defined only with great difficulty. Recent years have witnessed an increase in concern with stress. Contemporary life is said to lead to stress, people work under greater pressure and stresses in families turn men and women to the bottle, whether it contains alcohol or tranquillisers. The availability of stress reduction programmes of varying quality is escalating, doctors are exhorted to help their patients with stress-related problems, be they physical or psychological, and doctors themselves are complaining ever more vociferously of the stresses they are under. But just what is stress and how can it be managed? One strategy is to eschew all attempt at definition and conduct controlled trials (Kiely & McPherson, 1986) or publish reports (Webb et al., 1988) to see if it, whatever it is, can be reduced. Another is to study the presumed results of stress. As discussed in Chapter 9, expressions like 'burnout' have been adopted to describe a syndrome of chronic frustration in the work place leading to lowered morale, neglect of normal responsibilities and a flattened, disinterested response to further stress (Maslach, 1982; Maslach & Jackson, 1981). Stress can also be regarded as the source of multiple physical problems, although defining the nature and degree of stress remains problematic, and the evidence for causal connections is often found wanting.

Arguably, a more useful approach is to break the concept down into its component parts (Levine & Ursin, 1991). There are the *input* or stress stimuli. These include all manner of negative physical, emotional or social events which impact on the person over varying lengths of time. The *processing systems*, which include the subjective experience of a stimulus as stressful or not, are a decisive intermediary. Style of coping, cognitive appraisal of events and the quality of social supports will each determine whether an event such as bereavement leads to physical or psychological morbidity. By coping is meant the ability of the individual to deal with, or reduce the impact of, the input. Over and above these processing systems, genetic, personality and age factors will all play a role in the *output* or stress responses which occur. These are the overt behavioural and physiological changes which can be observed by the individual or outside observers. There is no overall consensus on the nature of the 'alarm' system or stress response which results in a generalised increase in arousal, mediated by the reticular formation in the brain (Levine & Ursin, 1991). Furthermore, there is little agreement on when such a reaction becomes maladaptive and damaging in itself. It is this process, however, with which we are most interested. Physiological responses which are part of the output may be used as indicators of whether stress is occurring and the degree of it. To be useful, however, a stress marker must be quantifiable and accurately measured. This operational approach to stress allows the component parts of the pathway to be tested or subjected to intervention, despite the disadvantage that many of the factors involved in the development of stress reactions are overlapping and confounding.

Stress responses must not be regarded as something always to be avoided. Clearly, they may be the driving force behind avoidance of damage or the action of problem-solving. Such responses are an essential part of the adaptation of the organism. Even unpleasant emotional states associated with stress may be required for full resolution of the problem. This is exemplified in the current approach to treatment of acute post-traumatic stress disorders, wherein patients are encouraged to expose themselves to mental images of the trauma in order to allow gradual resolution of the experience (Turner, 1992).

Stress and the immune system

Stress is postulated to cause changes in the immune system which may lead to infectious, neoplastic or autoimmune disease. Why stress should lead to *diminished* immune function rather than increased efforts to safeguard the organism is often not addressed. The implicit assumption behind much of this work is that stress is a factor which overwhelms the system and leads to decompensation. In HIV infection it is proposed that physiological responses in an already compromised immune system might further reduce immune competence and lead to the appearance of HIV disease. The immune system is a complicated, interdependent system by which the body recognises and protects itself against foreign material, particularly micro-organisms, viruses and cancerous cells. This is not the place for a detailed discussion of the immune system, and the reader is advised to consult a suitable text. The field is highly specialised and, particularly with the impetus of AIDS research, is in a state of flux. In brief, the system is based on humoral and cellular components and is broadly enhancing or suppressive in function. In the humoral system, there is a complex relationship between T- and B-lymphocytes and macrophages. T-lymphocyte helper cells which carry the genetic marker CD4 recognise and attach to an antigen, present it to the B-lymphocyte which undergoes a morphological transformation to become a plasma cell. The plasma cell produces and secretes specific antibodies which neutralise or destroy the antigen. Antibodies will also attach to larger antigens and allow another cell in the immune system, the macrophage, to engulf and destroy them. T-suppressor lymphocytes, which carry the genetic marker CD8, act to down-regulate and thereby to control the proliferative responses. Various classes of antibodies or immunoglobulins are produced by B-lymphocytes, after transformation, and these classes function at specific sites in the body. For example, immunoglobulin A concentrates in body fluids, and is active specifically at mucosal surfaces, protecting the body from invasion by foreign antigens. The cellular immune response is composed of so-called killer cells which seek out and destroy foreign material. These are a form of T-lymphocyte which are also dependent on T-helper cells for proliferation. Natural killer cells are lymphocytes which act in a non-specific fashion and do not seem to require transformation or sensitisation by T-helper cells in order to act against antigens. They can be identified in the blood using specific fluorescent, monoclonal antibodies. Loss of natural killer cell function renders the body vulnerable to infection by viruses, and diminishes resistance to neoplastic proliferation. Both humoral and cellular systems are subject to regulation by lymphokines, such as interleukins and interferons, which are humoral factors released by T-lymphocytes and macrophages. Autoimmune diseases occur when there is a failure of immune regulation at either cellular or humoral level, and the body fails to distinguish between foreign and native material. Self-directed immune responses may result and are observed in disorders such as rheumatoid arthritis.

There is an intimate and interdependent relationship between the CNS, hypothalamus–pituitary–adrenal axis and immune system. The function of the CNS is analogous to the immune system in discriminating between self and non-self and in protecting the integrity of the self against intrusions of non-self (Perez & Farrant, 1988). The immune system and CNS also share the crucial function of memory. Receptors for neurohormones occur on lymphocytes and many hormones are able to influence lymphocytic function (Perez & Farrant, 1988). The autonomic nervous system, which is sensitive to changes in psychological arousal, supplies several organs important in immune function such as the thymus and spleen. It has even been claimed that specific responses in the autonomic system may be linked to several basic emotional states such as anger or joy (Ekman, Levenseon & Friesen, 1983).

The many problems involved in exploring links between psychological and immunological factors explain why little definitive research has been published. Immunological tests are expensive to perform and may be difficult to interpret, there is little understanding of the time relationship between input (stressor) and immunological reaction, links between immunological change and disease outcome are poorly understood, and there are long delays in conducting appropriate prospective studies (Temoshok, 1988). Most work to date has been of a cross-sectional nature in which various psychological and social variables have been studied in relation to immune function. There have been reports of reduced immune function with dysphoric mood states, immunosuppressive behaviours such as substance abuse, adverse life experiences and vulnerability (Kaplan, 1991). By the latter is intended a lack of coping ability or 'hardiness' of personality and the absence of social support. Many studies have been handicapped by use of diverse measures of psychological and social function, a failure to take account of the impact and salience of the stressor for the individual, and a lack of concordance between psychosocial function and immune factor (Kaplan, 1991).

Bereavement and immune function

The clearest evidence linking immunity with stress comes from studies of bereavement, perhaps due to the presumption that loss of a spouse or long-term partner is one of the most severe life experiences. It has been demonstrated that death of a spouse or close family member may impair both humoral and cell-mediated immunity in the bereaved (Bartrop, 1977; Schleifer et al., 1989; Linn, Linn & Jenson, 1982). Although lymphocyte counts do not change, alterations in their responses to mitogen stimulation occur for between 4 and 14 months after bereavement. Linn et al. (1982) also made the observation that abnormal lymphocyte responses were more common in bereaved subjects who were significantly depressed. Irwin et al. (1990) went further in a controlled, prospective study of three groups of women, in one of which their husbands were dying of lung cancer, the second of which the husbands had died, and the third in which the husbands were in good health. Natural killer cell activity was reduced in women who had made poorer social adjustments as measured by a standardised rating scale. Loss of T-suppressor cells, an increase in the ratio of T-helper to T-suppressor cells and reduced natural killer cell activity, were correlated with higher scores on the Hamilton Depression Rating Scale. It must be stressed, however, that, although significant changes were noted, cell counts remained in the normal range, and it was not possible to gauge their effects on health outcome.

Depression and immunity

Mood changes associated with Cushing disease and iatrogenic steroids are well recognised, as are the changes in cortisol secretion during severe depression. There have been many studies investigating links between mood, the hypothalamus–pituitary–adrenal axis and the immune system. However, use of differing measures of immune function in a rapidly evolving field makes interpretation and comparison of results difficult. In evaluating the importance of these studies, it is important to clarify the questions posed (Hickie et al., 1990). Since changes in immune function may be state dependent, only *current* depressed mood should be considered. Severity of depressed mood and particularly 'endogenous' depression in which markers of CNS disregulation, such as shortened rapid eye movement (REM) sleep latency, and hypothalamic–pituitary dysfunction occur, are also likely to be important in the search for links between immune function and depression.

In the largest study yet reported, Schleifer et al. (1989) found no important differences in humoral or cell-mediated immunity between 91 unmedicated patients with major depressive disorder and matched controls. The sample contained mainly young outpatients. However, in a more recent, controlled study of 44 depressed men and women, most of whom were inpatients and all of whom were under the age of 47 years Evans et al. (1992), reported significant reductions in cell-mediated immunity in men. Depressed males had lower Leu-11 counts (cells carrying the CD16 marker, all of which have potential natural killer cell activity (NKA)), NKA and Leu-7 lymphocytes (some of which have NKA) than male controls, while there were no differences between depressed women and controls on all three measures. The authors postulated that women may be more resistant to immune dysfunction under stress than men, and cited other evidence that suggests that women have lower cortisol and systolic blood pressure responses to stress. They also acknowledged, however, that a type II error was possible in their female group owing either to smaller numbers or possible confounding effects of the menstrual cycle. Although severity of depression was not directly associated with NKA, there was some evidence that reductions in NK cell numbers and killing capacity were related to severity.

Both Schleifer et al. (1989) and Evans et al. (1992) enlisted young, depressed patients. In a review of controlled studies of major depression in mainly hospitalised patients, Hickie et al. (1990) calculated that the mean age of patients in studies reporting some significant effect on immune function in depressives was almost ten years higher than in those which failed to find differences between depressives and controls. The mean age of patients shown to have disordered immune function is similar to that typically reported for patients with endogenous depression. It remains unclear whether age and severity are independent determinants of impaired immune function or whether endogenous depression, which typically occurs in older subjects, is the most crucial factor. Age itself is known to lead to changes in immune function and hence carefully controlled comparisons are essential. Finally, it remains to be established whether immune dysfunction measured in depressed patients has any significant clinical consequences. There is indirect evidence that patients with major psychiatric syndromes have higher rates of physical illness and death (independent of self-harm or suicide) (Kendler, 1986) and that well-demarcated depressive syndromes in people aged over 55 years are associated with a fourfold increase of death from natural causes (Bruce & Leaf, 1989). However, substance abuse, poor socioeconomic conditions, and dietary neglect, are factors common to populations of psychiatric patients, and may have confounding effects on overall morbidity and mortality. To date, there are no empirical data to indicate that stress or depression-related alterations in immune function, such as NKA, are related to the development, or course, of physical disease (Evans et al., 1992).

Immunity in other serious illnesses

There is a considerable body of research on the role of stress, immunity and the development and progression of other disorders. Again, evidence as to the role of psychological factors in development and prognosis of the illness is conflicting. Study of emotional and immune factors in disorders other than AIDS is somewhat more straightforward, however, as the immune system itself is presumed not to be centrally involved. Although links have been reported between stress, certain personality types, and the development of cancer, it is quite unclear whether, or how, this is mediated through the immune system (Fletcher, 1991). The effect of psychological factors on the subsequent course of cancers has also received intensive study, but with no overall consensus. Cooper and Watson (1991) provide an excellent, up-to-date review of the influence of emotions, personality and stress on the development and course of malignant disease.

Psychological and social influences on immunity in HIV infection

What answers do we have to questions concerning stress and immune function in HIV infection? Do social or psychological stresses such as discrimination, rejection, depression and bereavement, accelerate deterioration of immune function and hasten the onset of HIV disease and, perhaps more importantly, does avoidance of, or appropriate responses to, such stress ameliorate the immunological effects? Unfortunately, simple correlations between progression of HIV infection and psychological distress do not allow us to decide which is causative.

Only work concentrating on specific immunological markers will be considered here. Further information about the effects of stress on disease progression which does not include an explicit immunological component is discussed in Chapter 3. Similar caveats to the conclusions from immunological research in bereavement and depression apply here, but with the added complication that immune function is already impaired in ways which are yet to be completely understood. It may not be possible to extrapolate findings from other populations to people with HIV infection in whom the immune system is already compromised and is perhaps significantly different in function and responsivity. Furthermore, studies of immune function and psychological health in HIV infection must take account of the possible immunosuppressive effects of alcohol and other substance abuse which are relatively common in affected populations.

In a review in the late 1980s, Temoshok (1988) concluded that, at that time, there were no published studies which unequivocally linked psychological and immunological variables to HIV disease outcome. What has occurred since then? While there have been many studies measuring differing parameters and often involving small sample sizes, only larger, well-conducted studies will be considered here. Although a range of immunological markers is employed in non-HIV, psycho-immunological work, CD4 counts and percentages are used more often in the AIDS field as they are the immune markers most closely allied to progression of HIV disease. None the less, other immune markers may be as, or more, important than CD4 lymphocytes. Unavoidably, in such a complex field, there have been conflicting findings.

Among studies giving rise to positive findings, Kemeny et al. (1990) reported that 35 chronically depressed, HIV-positive men had steeper declines in CD4 cell percentages over two years than 70 comparison, non-depressed, seropositive, control men. Significantly fewer of the depressed men showed a flattened (plateau) period in CD4 decline over a five-year period than the non-depressed. Antoni et al. (1990) reported that, in gay men undergoing HIV testing, immunological changes consequent on stress may be altered. Forty-six, healthy, homosexual men underwent a range of immunological, endocrine and psychological measures, taken at six time points over a ten-week observation period in the middle of which serostatus was notified. Only men who were found subsequently to be HIV negative were reported on, as the aim was to monitor changes in healthy men. T-cell proliferative responses to antigen stimulation were depressed, while cortisol levels were elevated at entry to the study. There were no changes in beta-endorphin levels throughout the ten-week period. A preference for a coping strategy of denial of the stress of HIV testing was associated with less immune suppression. Higher baseline cortisol levels, and lower denial coping strategy scores, were associated with the most impaired immune proliferative responses at study entry. Furthermore, there was a positive association between intrusiveness of thoughts concerning future risk of AIDS and plasma cortisol levels at all three *post-notification* points, despite the fact that all subjects had been notified that they were HIV seronegative. It is difficult to interpret this study. The authors add, in a footnote to their paper, that 25 additional men recruited to the study, and later found to be seropositive, were not included in the analysis because they already demonstrated blunted lymphocyte proliferative responses. It appears that they were only interested in healthy gay men undergoing stress. Why HIV testing was chosen as the specific stressor is therefore not completely clear. Perhaps it was chosen as a major stressor of similar impact to all the men involved. Unfortunately, by using a volunteer sample in a study associated with HIV testing, one runs the risk of including many men who are overly concerned about their risk of infection. The persistent concerns about AIDS after notification of a negative result indicates that this may well have been a factor here. A control group not undergoing testing would have been a useful addition to the study.

Many well-conducted studies have been unable to establish that psychological or social factors have important, measurable effects on immune function in HIV infection. In a prospective study over three months, Perry et al. (1991) correlated psychosocial factors with total CD4 counts in men and women from various risk groups. Although there were some cross-sectional associations between CD4 cells and state anxiety, or death of a spouse or close sexual partner in the preceding two years, none of the psychological or social factors measured at baseline was predictive of CD4 cell counts three months later. The authors were careful to control for baseline immune measures in their analysis. Gorman et al. (1991), reported on 24-hour urinary-free cortisol levels and lymphocyte counts in a longitudinal study of 112 well, seropositive, homosexual men matched with 75 seronegative, homosexual men. No significant correlation was found between urinary-free cortisol and any current DSMIIIR Axis I diagnosis, although there were small, but significant, correlations between 24-hour urinary-free cortisol and levels of anxiety and depression in the seropositive group. More importantly, however, there was no relationship between cortisol level and the number of CD4 or CD8 lymphocytes or CD4/CD8 ratio. There were several limitations to the study which may have increased the likelihood of negative findings. Although intended as a controlled, longitudinal study of physical, psychological and neurological functioning in HIV infection, data on cortisol levels were cross-sectional in nature. Overall, levels of psychopathology in the study population were low and, while it is possible that lymphocyte function is affected by cortisol levels, only the number, rather than the function, of T-lymphocytes was measured.

In a three-year prospective study of initially well, seronegative, homosexual men, Kessler et al. (1991) found no significant association between stressful life events, including numbers of lovers, friends and acquaintances who were diagnosed with AIDS, or had died with AIDS, and drop in CD4 cells. However, the authors acknowledged that a trend existed for a drop in CD4 cells in men suffering stressful life events which might have reached statistical significance in a larger sample. Rabkin et al. (1991) correlated CD4 and CD8 subsets and HIV signs and symptoms with psychiatric diagnoses, psychiatric symptoms and psychosocial stressors, in a six-month prospective study of 124 seropositive homosexual men. Subjects were part of a five year cohort study of factors affecting progression of HIV infection. They were a well-educated, professional group who were financially secure. As well as the Structured Clinical Interview to make a DSMIIIR diagnosis (SCID) (Spitzer et al., 1988), subjects completed several standardised, self-report scales measuring levels of anxiety, depression, grief, demoralisation and hopelessness. Assessments were also made of life events and social conflict. At baseline, only ten men (8 per cent), had a current depressive disorder, of whom only five had a major depression, a level not significantly different to community samples. Furthermore, self-reported depressive symptoms, global distress and perceived stressors declined significantly in the study population over the six months. Men who were depressed, distressed, or who reported more life stressors, had no greater immunosuppression than others at baseline or at six months. Limitations acknowledged by the authors were the low prevalence and incidence of psychiatric problems and hence the reduced power of the study, the difficulty of deciding upon appropriate lengths of follow-up, the relatively early HIV stage of participants, and the possible insensitivity of T-cell subsets as measures of immune function. The final point is perhaps the most important. It seems inherently unlikely that overall immune function *in vivo* is directly related to T-cell numbers.

Finally, a recent study by Perry et al. (1992) has also drawn negative conclusions. In a study of a cohort of seropositive men, data on lymphocyte subsets and psychosocial measures were reported for 173 subjects at six months and 92 subjects at one year. Although some of the men had vague HIV-related symptoms at entry, none met criteria for stage 4A disease and none was taking HIV-related medications. By the end of follow-up, 4 per cent had received zidovudine. Standardised psychosocial variables showed no relationship with lymphocyte subsets either concurrently or prospectively. Cross-sectional correlations among 22 psychosocial variables and CD4 and CD8 counts and CD4/CD8 ratios were very low and remained minimal over the follow-up period. As the authors acknowledged, it is possible that the follow-up period was too short to detect possible relationships, although medical illnesses and treatments confound longer periods of follow-up. Perhaps the biggest caution in interpreting this study lies in the measures of immune function used. Although they involved cell counts which are often used to monitor the progression of HIV disease, such measures may be insufficient to detect more subtle changes in immune structure and function in this disorder. In any case, the authors warned clinicians against recommending that patients reduce their stress levels in the hope of sustaining their T-cells, out of concern that such a stance may foster self-accusation when physical symptoms do occur.

Intervention

Even if immunity is impaired by psychological distress, will intervention to reduce that stress improve immune function, or slow further deterioration? At least one study has attempted to address this issue. Coates et al. (1989) carried out an eight week stress reduction programme with 64 volunteer, seropositive homosexual men. Men selected were those who were in good health and not practising regular meditation. Half were randomised to a stress reduction programme consisting of two hours weekly for eight weeks, in which they were taught systematic relaxation, 'healthy habit change', and skills for managing stress. Immunological tests included T-cell subset counts, NKA and lymphocyte proliferative activity. Although it was reported that the men in the stress reduction group significantly reduced their numbers of sexual partners, markers of immune function showed no significant differences between the groups. Changes in psychological functioning were not reported. Although the results are negative, there were several problems with the study. Baseline levels of emotional distress between the two groups are not reported. Single measures of immune function at entry and following treatment may not be sensitive enough to detect change. The stress reduction intervention may not have been efficacious but, without data on the levels of stress and psychological functioning throughout the trial, this is impossible to gauge. Finally, the authors raise the intriguing possibility that since the second test for immune function was taken four days after the ending of the group, immune responses may have temporarily regressed because of sadness at leaving the group. Again, in the absence of psychological data, this possibility cannot be examined.

Clinical relevance

How does this work inform us in our approach to patients? Many people with HIV infection and AIDS seek alternative treatments in the belief that they will boost their immune system. Some of these treatments are psychological in nature and involve relaxation, self-hypnosis and meditation, and cognitive inducement of the immune system. In the latter, patients will focus on imagery of their immune system, particularly on the cellular components which are most readily understood, in an attempt to boost it positively. This stems from popular beliefs that a 'fighting spirit' will prevent worsening of their clinical status. As discussed, although empirical evidence for unequivocal effects on the immune system are lacking, there is usually little to be gained from discouraging patients in these pursuits. Our level of knowledge is simply not secure enough for us to declare that such pursuits are a waste of time and money. None the less, judicious help to ensure that patients are not exploited may be necessary. It may also be necessary for AIDS physicians and nurses to decide how far they can go in endorsing patients in their attempts to manipulate the immune system by alternative psychological and medical methods, particularly if traditional therapies are foregone and patients' health is placed in greater danger (Gorman & Kertzner, 1990). For the mental health worker, it may be sufficient to be aware of the principal ways in which people with HIV infection seek to boost their immunity, and to incorporate this into their therapeutic alliance with them. There is little to gain from either ridicule or over-endorsement of unsubstantiated claims.

Conclusions

There is now a large body of work correlating markers of immune function with psychological states, particularly with depression, bereavement and other reactions to stress. Studies have been hampered by our rudimentary understanding of the enormously complicated and interdependent immune and central nervous systems. Stressors are difficult to define or measure, and many people with HIV infection are subject to multiple, interwoven stressors, all of which may have confounding influences on each other. Individual factors such as coping style and personality may also confound simple comparisons.

Even if stressors can be identified by an outside observer, their impact may not be clear. How do emotional expression or denial under the same stressor differ in their effects on immune function? There has often been a confusion between immune structure and function and a lack of attention to the significance of *in vitro* abnormalities. Nor have links always been established between demonstrable changes in immune function and disease status. The degree of immune impairment needed, before emotional stress might show an effect, is an unknown, but possibly critical, factor in such work.

Despite popular belief on the part of patients and some of their carers, the evidence in HIV infection that psychological or social factors have an important influence on immune competence, or on progression of the disorder, remains to be clearly demonstrated. Although emotional factors may have direct effects on neurohormone release and on immune response, the relationships are complicated and do not allow simple explanations of the direct influence of stress on immune function or vice versa. There is some evidence linking stressful life events with an elevated risk of illness onset in previously well HIV-seropositive men, but careful prospective work correlating psychological and social variables with CD4 lymphocyte counts has not established any direct association. Although it is not yet possible to attribute disease progression to the direct effects of emotional distress on the immune system, extensive work is under way to examine these issues further. Until unequivocal evidence is established that stress impairs immune function in HIV infection, there is a danger that published half truths will lead patients to forego established treatments in favour of unproven psychological or physical treatments which they believe might boost their immune function more effectively.

REFERENCES

Abed, R. T. & Neira-Munoz, E. (1990). A survey of general practitioners' opinions and attitudes to drug addicts and addiction. *British Journal of Addiction*, **85**, 131–6

a'Brook, M. K. (1967). Psychiatric illness in the medical profession. *British Journal of Psychiatry*, **113**, 1013–23.

Adib, S. M., Joseph, J. G., Ostrow, D. G. & James, S. A. (1991). Predictors of relapse in sexual practices among homosexual men. *AIDS Education and Prevention*, **3**, 293–304.

Adib, S. M. & Ostrow, D. G. (1991). Trends in HIV/AIDS behavioural research among homosexual and bisexual men in the United States: 1981–1991. *AIDS Care*, **3**:3, 281–7.

Adler, M. W. (1987). Patient safety and doctors with HIV infection. *British Medical Journal*, **295**, 1297–8.

AIDS Group of the United Kingdom Haemophilia Centre Directors with the Co-operation of the United Kingdom Haemophilia Centre Directors. (1988). Prevalence of antibody to HIV in haemophiliacs in the United Kingdom: a second survey. *Clinical Laboratories in Haemotology*, **10**, 187–91

Allebeck, P. & Bolund, C. (1991). Suicides and suicide attempts in cancer patients. *Psychological Medicine*, **21**, 979–84.

Allen, S., Tice, J., Van de Perre, P., Serufilira, A., Hudes, E., Nsengumuremyi, F., Bogaerts, J., Lindan, C. & Hulley, S. (1992). Effect of serotesting with counselling on condom use and seroconversion among HIV discordant couples in Africa. *British Medical Journal*, **304**, 1605–9.

Alloway, R. & Bebbington, P. (1987). The buffer theory of social support – a review of the literature. *Psychological Medicine*, **17**, 91–108.

American Medical Association Council on Ethical and Judicial Affairs (1992). Decisions near the end of life. *Journal of the American Medical Association*, **267**, 2229–33.

American Psychiatric Association (1987). *Diagnostic and Statistical Manual – Third Edition Revised*. Washington DC: American Psychiatric Association.

American Psychiatric Association Ad Hoc Committee on AIDS Policy (1988*a*). AIDS policy: guidelines for inpatient psychiatric units. *American Journal of Psychiatry*, **145**, 542.

American Psychiatric Association Ad Hoc Committee on AIDS Policy (1988*b*). AIDS policy: confidentiality and disclosure. *American Journal of Psychiatry*, **145**, 541.

American Psychiatric Association Commission on AIDS (1992*a*). AIDS policy: guidelines for inpatient psychiatric units. *American Journal of Psychiatry*, **149**, 722.

American Psychiatric Association Commission on AIDS (1992*b*). AIDS policy: guidelines for outpatient psychiatic services. *American Journal of Psychiatry*, **149**, 721.

Ancelle-Park, R. (1993). Expanded European AIDS case definition. *Lancet*, **341**, 441.

Anderson, J. (1990). AIDS in Thailand. *British Medical Journal* **300**, 415–16

Anderson, P. & Mayon-White, R. (1988). General practitioners and management of infection with HIV. *British Medical Journal*, **296**, 535–7.

Anon. (1964). Suicide among doctors. *British Medical Journal*, **i**, 789–90.

Anon. (1985). Retaining patients with AIDS. *British Medical Journal*, **291**, 1102.

Anon. (1987). AIDS, HIV and general practice. *Journal of the Royal College of General Practitioners*, **37**, 289–90.

Anon. (1991). Your heroin, sir. *Lancet*, **337**, 402.

Antoni, M. H., August, S., LaPerriere, A., Bagget, L., Klimas, N., Ironson, G., Schneiderman, N. & Fletcher, M. A. (1990). Psychological and neuroendocrine measures related to functional immune changes in anticipation of HIV-1 serostatus notification. *Psychosomatic Medicine*, **52**, 496–510.

Arana, G. W. (1982). The impaired physician. *General Hospital Psychiatry*, **4**, 147–53.

Aruffo, J. F., Coverdale, J. H., Chacko, R. C. & Dworkin, R. J. (1990). Knowledge about AIDS among women psychiatric outpatients. *Hospital and Community Psychiatry*, **41**(3), 326–8.

Asher, R. (1951). Munchausen's syndrome. *Lancet*, **i**, 339–41.

Ashurst, P. M. (1981). *Counselling in General Practice. Report to the Mental Health Foundation Conference*, London: Mental Health Foundation.

Atkinson Jr, J. H., Grant, I., Kennedy, C. J., Richman, D. D., Spector, S. A. & McCutchan, J. A. (1988). Prevalence of psychiatric disorders among men infected with human immunodeficiency virus. *Archives of General Psychiatry*, **45**, 859–64.

Baer, J. W., Hall, J. M., Holm, K. & Lewitter-Koehler, S. (1987). Challenges in developing an inpatient psychiatric program for patients with AIDS and ARC. *Hospital and Community Psychiatry*, **38**, 1299–303.

Baer, J. W. (1989). Study of 60 patients with AIDS or AIDS-related complex requiring psychiatric hospitalization. *American Journal of Psychiatry*, **146**(10), 1285–8.

Bagnall, G., Plant, M. & Warwick, W. (1990). Alcohol, drugs and AIDS-related risks: results from a prospective study. *AIDS Care*, **2**(4), 309–17.

Bailey, J. T., Stefen, S. M. & Grout, J. W. (1980). The stress audit: identifying the stressors of ICU nursing. *Journal of Nursing Education*, **19**, 15–25.

Barczak, P., Kane, N., Andrews, S., Congdon, A. M., Clay, J. C., & Betts, T. (1988). Patterns of psychiatric morbidity in a genito-urinary clinic. *British Journal of Psychiatry*, **152**, 698–700.

Bartrop, R. W., Lazarus, I., Luckhurst, E., Kiloh, L. G. & Penny, R. (1977). Depressed lymphocyte function after bereavement. *Lancet*, **i**, 834–6

Baur, S. (1988). *Hypochondria: Woeful Imaginings*. Berkeley, University of California Press.

Bayer, R. (1990). AIDS and the future of reproductive freedom. *Milbank Quarterly*, **68**(2), 179–204.

Beck, E. J., Donegan, C., Cohen, C. S., Moss, V. & Terry, P. (1990). An update on HIV testing at a London STD clinic: long-term impact on the AIDS media campaigns. *Genitourinary Medicine*, **66**, 142–7.

Becker, M. H. & Joseph, J. G. (1988). AIDS and behavioural change to reduce risk: a review. *American Journal of Public Health*, **78**(4), 394–410.

Bell, G., Cohen, J. & Cremona, A. (1990). How willing are GPs to manage drug misuse? *Health Trends*, **22**, 56–7.

Beltangady, M. (1988). The risk of suicide in persons with AIDS. *Journal of the American Medical Association*, **260**(1), 29.

Bennett, L., Michie, P. & Kippax, S. (1991). Quantitative analysis of burnout and its associated factors in AIDS nursing. *AIDS Care*, **3**, 181–92.

Berger, R. M. (1990). Men together: understanding the gay couple. *Journal of Homosexuality*, **19**, 31–49.

Bewley, S. (1988). Who defaults after treatment for gonorrhoea? Randomised controlled study of effect of an educational leaflet. *Genitourinary Medicine*, **64**, 241–44.

Bhanji, S. & Mahony, J. D. H. (1978). The value of a psychiatric service within the venereal disease clinic. *British Journal of Venereal Diseases*, **54**, 266–8.

Bhugra, D. & King, M. B. (1989). Controlled comparison of attitudes of psychiatrists, general practitioners, homosexual doctors amd homosexual men to homosexuality. *Journal of the Royal Society of Medicine*, **82**, 603–5.

Binder, R. L. (1987). AIDS antibody tests on inpatient psychiatric units. *American Journal of Psychiatry*, **144**, 176–81.

Bird, A. G. (1988). HIV infection: the Swedish approach. *Journal of the Royal College of Physicians of London*, **22**, 114–17.

Bird, A. G., Gore, S. M., Leigh-Brown, A. J. & Carter, D. C. (1991). Escape from collective denial: HIV transmission during surgery. *British Medical Journal*, **303**, 351–2.

Black, D. (1987). Doctors with HIV infection. *British Medical Journal*, **295**, 1345.

Blaney, N. T., Goodkin, K., Morgan, R. O., Feaster, D., Millon, C., Szapocznik, J. & Eisdorfer, C. (1991). A stress-moderator model of distress in early HIV-1 infection: concurrent analysis of life events, hardiness and social support. *Journal of Psychosomatic Research*, **35**(2/3), 297–305.

Blomqvist, V., Jonsson, L. & Theorell, T. (1991). Life events and coping patterns reported in HIV-infected haemophiliacs a year after diagnosis. *Scandinavian Journal of Social Medicine*, **19**(2), 94–8.

Bloor, M. J., McKeganey, N. P., Finlay, A. & Barnard, M. A. (1992). The inappropriateness of psycho-social models of risk behaviour for understanding HIV-related risk practices among Glasgow male prostitutes. *AIDS Care*, **4**(2), 131–7.

Blumenfeld, M., Smith, P. J., Milazzo, J. (1987). Survey of attitudes of nurses working with AIDS patients. *General Hospital Psychiatry*, **9**, 58–63.

Boccellari, A. A. & Dilley, J. W. (1992). Management and residential placement problems of patients with HIV-related cognitive impairment. *Hospital and Community Psychiatry*, **43**, 32–7.

Bor, R., Perry, L., Miller, R. & Jackson, J. (1989). Strategies for counselling the 'worried well' in relation to AIDS: discussion paper. *Journal of the Royal Society of Medicine*, **82**, 218–20.

Boyd, J. S., Kerr, S., Maw, R. D., Finnigan, E. A. & Kilbane, P. K. (1990). Knowledge of HIV infection and AIDS and attitudes to testing and counselling among general practitioners in Northern Ireland. *British Journal of General Practice*, **40**, 158–60.

Boyton, R. & Scambler, G. (1988). Survey of general practitioners' attitudes to AIDS in the North West Thames and East Anglian regions. *British Medical Journal*, **296**, 538–40.

Bradbeer, C. (1987). HIV and sexual lifestyle. *British Medical Journal*, **294**, 5–6.

Bradbeer, C. (1989). Mothers with HIV. *British Medical Journal*, **299**, 806–7.

Bredfeldt, R. C., Dardeau, F. M., Wesley, R. M., Vaughan-Wrobel, B. C. & Markland, L. (1991). AIDS: family physicians' attitudes and experiences. *Journal of Family Practice*, **32**, 71–5.

Breitbart, W. & Knight, R. T. (1988). AIDS and neuroleptic malignant syndrome. *Lancet*, **ii**, 1488–9.

Bresolin, L. B., Rinaldi, R. C., Henning, J. J., Harvey, L. K., Hendee, W. R. & Schwarz, R. (1990). Attitudes of US primary care physicians about HIV disease and AIDS. *AIDS Care*, **2**, 117–25.

Brettle, R. P. (1987). Drug abuse and human immunodeficiency virus infection in Scotland. *Journal of the Royal Society of Medicine*, **80**, 274–8.

Brettle, R. P. (1990). Hospital health care for HIV infection with particular reference to injecting drug users. *AIDS Care*, **2**, 171–81.

Brewer, T. F. & Derrickson, J. (1992). AIDS in prison: a review of epidemiology and preventive policy. *AIDS*, **6**, 623–8.

British Association of Counselling. (1979) *Counselling: Definition of Terms in Use with Expansion and Rationale*. Rugby, England: British Association of Counselling.

Brown, G. R. & Rundell, J. R. (1990). Prospective study of psychiatric morbidity in HIV-seropositive women without AIDS. *General Hospital Psychiatry*, **12**, 30–5.

Brown, G. W. & Harris, T. (1978). *Social Origins of Depression. A Study of Psychiatric Disorder in Women*. London: Tavistock.

Bruce, M. L. & Leaf, P. J. (1989). Psychiatric disorders and 15 month mortality. *American Journal of Public Health*, **79**, 727–30.

Bucknall, A. (1986). Regional patterns of AIDS and HIV infection. *Journal of the Royal College of General Practitioners*, **292**, 491–2.

Buhrich, N. & Cooper, D. A. (1987). Requests for psychiatric consultation concerning 22 patients with AIDS and ARC. *Australian and New Zealand Journal of Psychiatry*, **21**, 346–53.

Buhrich, N., Cooper, D. A. & Freed, E. (1988). HIV infection associated with symptoms indistinguishable from functional psychosis. *British Journal of Psychiatry*, **152**, 649–53.

Busch, K. (1989). Psychotic states in human immunodeficiency virus illness. *Current Opinion in Psychiatry*, **2**, 3–6.

Campbell, C. A. (1990). Prostitution and AIDS. In D. G. Ostrow (Ed.), *Behavioural Aspects of AIDS* New York: Plenum.

Caputi, C. & King, M. B. (1992). *Prevalence and risk factors for psychiatric morbidity in HIV infection in São Paulo, Brazil.* Paper presented at the VIIIth International Conference on AIDS, Amsterdam.

Carballo, M. & Miller, D. (1989). HIV counselling: problems and opportunities in defining the new agenda for the 1990s. *AIDS Care*, **1**, 17–23.

Carne, C. A., Stibe, C., Bronkhurst, A., Newman, S. P., Weller, I. V. D., Kendall, B. E. & Harrison, M. J. G. (1989). Subclinical neurological and neuropsychological effect of infection with HIV. *Genitourinary Medicine*, **65**, 151–6.

Carvell, A. L. M. & Hart, G. J. (1990). Risk behaviours for HIV infection among drug users in prison. *British Medical Journal* **300**, 1383–4.

Catalan, J. (1990). *Psychiatric problems in HIV infected men with haemophilia.* Presented at the Conference on Neurology and Psychiatry of AIDS, Monterey, California, June 16–19.

Catalan, J., Bradley, M., Gallwey, J. & Hawton, K. (1981). Sexual dysfunction and psychiatric morbidity in patients attending a clinic for sexually transmitted diseases. *British Journal of Psychiatry*, **138**, 292–6.

Catalan, J., Klimes, I., Bond, A., Day, A., Garrod, A. & Rizza, C. (1992). The psychosocial impact of HIV infection in men with haemophilia: controlled investigation and factors associated with psychiatric morbidity. *Journal of Psychosomatic Research*, **36**, 409–16.

Catalan, J., Klimes, I., Bond, A., Garrod, A., Day, A. & Rizza, C. (1989). *Psychosocial and neurological status of haemophiliacs and gay men with HIV infection: a controlled investigation.* Presented at the Vth International Conference on AIDS, Montreal Canada, Book of abstracts ThBP.31, International Development Research Centre, Canada.

Catalan, J., Riccio, M. & Thompson, C. (1989). HIV disease and psychiatric practice. *Psychiatric Bulletin*, **13**, 316–32.

Cave, D. (1983). Bereavement and the unmarried partner. Bereavement care. *Cruse*, summer.

Centers for Disease Control. (1987). Revision of the CDC surveillance case definition for acquired immunodeficiency syndrome. *MMWR*, **36**(15),

Chaava, T. (1990). Approaches to counselling in a Zambian rural community. *AIDS Care*, **2**, 81–7.

Chin, J. (1990). Current and future dimensions of the HIV/AIDS pandemic in women and children. *Lancet*, **336**, 221–4.

Chuang, H. T., Devins, G. M., Hunsley, J. & Gill, M. J. (1989). Psychosocial distress and well being among gay and bisexual men with human immunodeficiency virus infection. *American Journal of Psychiatry*, **146**, 876–80.

Chuang, H. T., Jason, G. W., Pajurkova, E. M. & Gill, M. J. (1992). Psychiatric morbidity in patients with HIV infection. *Canadian Journal of Psychiatry*, **37**, 109–15.

Clifford, D. B., Jacoby, R. G., Miller, J. P., Seyfried, W. R. & Glicksman, M. (1990). Neuropsychometric performance of asymptomatic HIV-infected individuals. *AIDS*, **4**, 767–74.

Coates, T. J., McKusick, L., Kuno, R. & Stites, D. P. (1989). Stress reduction training changed number of sexual partners but not immune function in men with HIV infection. *American Journal of Public Health*, **79**, 885–7.

Cochran, S. D. & Peplau, A. L. (1991). Sexual risk reduction behaviours among young heterosexual adults. *Social Science and Medicine*, **33**, 25–36.

Cohen, S. E., Mundy, T., Karassik, B., Lieb, L., Ludwig, D. D. & Ward, J. (1991). Neuropsychological functioning in human immunodeficiency virus type 1 seropositive children infected through neonatal blood transfusion. *Pediatrics*, **88**, 58–68.

Collier, D. J. & Beales, I. L. (1989). Drinking among medical students: a questionnaire survey. *British Medical Journal*, **299**, 19–22.

Commonwealth AIDS Research Grant Committee Working Party, (1990). Attitudes, knowledge and behaviour of general practitioners in relation to HIV infection and AIDS. *Medical Journal of Australia*, **153**, 5–12.

Condini, A., Axia, G., Cattelan, C., D'Urso, M. R., Laverda, A. M., Viero, F. & Zacchello, F. (1991). Development of language in 18–30 month old HIV-infected but not ill children. *AIDS*, **5**, 735–9.

Conwell, Y. & Caine, E. D. (1991). Rational suicide and the right to die. *New England Journal of Medicine*, **325**, 1100–3.

Cooke, M. (1986). Ethical issues in the care of patients with AIDS. *Quarterly Review Bulletin*, **12**, 343–6.

Cooper, C. L. & Watson,M. (1991). *Cancer and Stress*. Chichester: John Wiley.

Coutinho, R. A., van Andel, R. L. M. & Rijsdijk, T. J. (1988). Role of male prostitutes in spread of sexually transmitted diseases and human immunodeficiency virus. *Genitourinary Medicine*, **64**, 207–8.

Coxon, A. P. M. & Carballo, M. (1989). Research on AIDS: behavioural perspectives. *AIDS*, **3**, 191–7.

Creed, F., Mayou, R. & Hopkins, A. (1992). *Medical Symptoms not Explained by Organic Disease*. London: Royal Colleges of Psychiatrists and Physicians.

Cummings, M. A., Rapaport, M. & Cummings, K. L. (1986). A psychiatric staff response to acquired immune deficiency syndrome. *American Journal of Psychiatry*, **143**, 682.

Curran, J. W., Lawrence, D. N., Jaffe, H., Kaplan, J. E., Zyla, L. D., Chamberland, M., Weinstein, R., Lui, K., Schonberger, L. B., Spira, T. J., Alexander, W. J., Swinger, G., Ammann, A., Solomon, S., Auerbach, D., Mildvan, D.,

Stoneburner, R., Jason, J. M., Haverkos, H. H. & Evatt, B. L. (1984). AIDS associated with transfusions. *New England Journal of Medicine*, **310**, 69–75.

Curran, L., McHugh, M. & Mooney, K. (1989). HIV counselling in prisons. *AIDS Care*, **1**, 11–25.

Curtis, J. L., Crummey, F. C., Baker, S. N., Foster, R. E., Khanyile, C. S. & Wilkins, R. (1989). HIV screening and counseling for intravenous drug abuse patients. *Journal of the American Medical Association*, **261**, 258–62.

Dardick, L. & Grady, K. E. (1980). Openness betwen gay persons and health professionals. *Annals of Internal Medicine*, **93**, 115–19.

Darko, D. F., McCutchan, J. A., Kripke, D. F., Gillin, J. C. & Golshan, S. (1992). Fatigue, sleep disturbance, disability, and indices of progression of HIV infection. *American Journal of Psychiatry*, **149**, 514–20.

Davey, T. & Green, J. (1991). The worried well: ten years of a new face for an old problem. *AIDS Care*, **3**(3), 289–93.

Day, S. (1988). Prostitute women and AIDS: anthropology. *AIDS*, **2**(6), 421–8.

Day, S., Wrad, H. & Harris, J. R. W. (1988). Prostitute women and public health. *British Medical Journal*, **297**, 1585.

Department of Health. (1991). *AIDS–HIV Infected Health Care Workers. Occupational Guidance for Health Care Workers, their Physicians and Employers*. London: HMSO.

Department of Health. (1992). *The Health of the Nation: A Strategy for Health in England*. London: HMSO.

Department of Health and Welsh Office, (1990). *Code of Practice*. London: HMSO.

Dew, M. A., Ragni, M. V. & Nimorwicz, P. (1990). Infection with human immunodeficiency virus and vulnerability to psychiatric distress. *Archives of General Psychiatry*, **47**, 737–44.

Dew, M. A., Ragni, M. V. & Nimorwicz, P. (1991). Correlates of psychiatric distress among wives of hemophiliac men with and without HIV infection. *American Journal of Psychiatry*, **148**, 1016–22.

Deykin, E. Y., Levy, J. C. & Wells, V. (1987). Adolescent depression, alcohol and drug abuse. *American Journal of Public Health*, **77**, 178–80.

Dilley, J. W., Ochitill, H. N., Perl, M. & Volberding, P. A. (1985). Findings in psychiatric consultations with patients with acquired immune deficiency syndrome. *American Journal of Psychiatry*, **142**, 82–6.

Dohrenwend, B. S. & Dohrenwend, B. P. (1981). *Stressful Life Events and Their Context*. New York: Neale Watson.

Dole, V. P. (1989). Methadone treatment and the acquired immunodeficiency syndrome epidemic. *Journal of the American Medical Association*, **262**, 1681–2.

Douglas, C. J., Kalman, C. M. & Kalman, T. P. (1985). Homophobia among physicians and nurses :an empirical study. *Hospital and Community Psychiatry*, **36**, 1309–11.

Douglas, R. B., Blanks, R., Crowther, A. & Scott, G. (1988). A study of stress in West Midlands firemen using ambulatory electrocardiograms. *Journal of Work and Stress*, **2**, 309–18.

Dreyer, E. B., Kaiser, P. K., Offermann, J. T. & Lipton, S. A. (1990). HIV-1 coat protein neurotoxicity prevented by calcium channel antagonists. *Science*, **248**, 364–7.

Dunbar, N., Perdices, M., Grunseit, A. & Cooper, D. A. (1992). Changes in neuropsychological performance of AIDS-related complex patients who progress to AIDS. *AIDS*, **6**, 691–700.

Dunne, F. J. (1989). Alcohol and the immune system. *British Medical Journal*, **298**, 543–4.

Dworkin, J., Albrecht, G. & Cooksey, J. (1991). Concern about AIDS among hospital physicians, nurses and social workers. *Social Science and Medicine*, **33**, 239–48.

Dye, S. & Isaacs, C. (1991). Intravenous drug misuse among prison inmates: implications for spread of HIV. *British Medical Journal*, **302**, 1506.

Dyer, C. (1987). Doctors and AIDS and the *News of the World*. *British Medical Journal*, **295**, 1339–40.

Dyer, C. (1989). Haemophiliacs sue British government. *British Medical Journal*, **299**, 700–1.

Dyer, C. (1990). Justice versus equity for haemophiliacs with AIDS. *British Medical Journal*, **301**, 776.

Egan, V. (1992). Neuropsychological aspects of HIV infection. *AIDS Care*, **4**, 3–10.

Egan, V. G., Crawford, J. R., Brettle, R. P. & Goodwin, G. M. (1990). The Edinburgh cohort of HIV-positive drug users: current intellectual function is impaired, but not due to early AIDS dementia complex. *AIDS*, **4**, 651–6.

Ekman, P., Levenseon, R. W. & Friesen, W. V. (1983). Autonomic nervous system activity distinguishes among emotions. *Science*, **221**, 1208–10.

Ekstrand, M. L. & Coates, T. J. (1990). Maintenance of safer sexual behaviours and predictors of risky sex: the San Franciso Men's Health Study. *American Journal of Public Health*, **80**, 973–7.

Ellis, D., Collis, I., & King, M. (1993). A controlled comparison of HIV and general medical referrals to a liaison psychiatry service. *AIDS Care* (in press).

Engelsman, E. I. (1991). Drug misuse and the Dutch. *British Medical Journal*, **302**, 484–5.

Epstein, R., Christie, M., Frankel, R., Rousseau, B. A. & Shields, C. (1993). Understanding fear of contagion among physicians who care for HIV patients. *Family Medicine* (in press).

Evans, B. A., McLean, K. A., Dawson, S. G., Teece, S. A., Bond, R. A., MacRae, K. D. & Thorp, R. W. (1989). Trends in sexual behaviour and risk factors for HIV infection among homosexual men, 1984–7. *British Medical Journal*, **298**, 215–18.

Evans, D. L., Folds, J. D., Petitto, J. M., Golden, R. N., Pederson, C. A., Corrigan, M., Gilmore, J. H., Silva, S. G., Quade, D. & Ozer, H. (1992). Circulating natural killer cell phenotypes in men and women with major depression. *Archives of General Psychiatry*, **49**, 388–95.

Everall, I. P., Luthert, P. J. & Lantos, P. L. (1991). Neuronal loss in the frontal cortex in HIV infection. *Lancet*, **337**, 1119–21.

Farrell, M. & Strang, J. (1991). Drugs, HIV, and prisons. *British Medical Journal*, **302**, 1477–8.

Faulstich, M. E. (1987). Psychiatric aspects of AIDS. *American Journal of Psychiatry*, **551**, 556.

Fell, M., Newman, S., Herns, M., Durrance, P., Manji, H., Connolly, S., MacAllister, R., Weller, I. & Harrison, M. (1991). *Serial assessment of mood and psychiatric state – changes over time and relation to neuropsychological assessment - the Middlesex MRC cohort study*. Paper presented to the VIIth International Conference on AIDS, Florence, Book of Abstracts M. B. 2042.

Fenton, T. W. (1987). Practical problems in the management of AIDS-related psychiatric disorder. *Journal of the Royal Society of Medicine*, **80**, 271–4.

Ferguson, B. & Tyrer, P. (1988). Classifying personality disorder. In P. Tyrer (Ed.), *Personality Disorders. Diagnosis, Management and Course* (pp. 12–32). London: Wright.

Fernandez, F. & Levy, J. K. (1990). Adjuvant treatment of HIV dementia with psychostimulants. In D. G. Ostrow (Ed.), *Behavioral Aspects of AIDS* (pp. 235–246). New York: Plenum.

Fife-Schaw, C. R. & Breakwell, G. M. (1992). Estimating sexual behaviour parameters in the light of AIDS: a review of recent UK studies of young people. *AIDS Care*, **4**, 187–201.

Firth-Cozens, J. (1987). Emotional distress in junior house officers. *British Medical Journal*, **295**, 533–6.

Flavin, D. K., Franklin, J. E. & Frances, R. J. (1986). The acquired immune deficiency syndrome (AIDS) and suicidal behaviour in alcohol-dependent homosexual men. *American Journal of Psychiatry*, **143**, 1440–2.

Fletcher, B. (1991). *Work, Stress, Disease and Life Expectancy*. Chichester: John Wiley.

Folstein, M. F., Folstein, S. E. & McHugh, P. R. (1975). 'Mini-mental state': a practical method of grading the cognitive state of patients for the clinician. *Journal of Psychiatric Research*, **12**, 189–98.

Forstein, M. (1984). AIDS anxiety in the 'worried well'. In S. E. Nichols & D. G. Ostrow (Eds.), *Acquired Immune Deficiency Syndrome* (pp. 50–60). Washington DC: American Psychiatric Press Inc.

Frances, R. J., Wikstrom, T. & Alcena, V. (1985). Contracting AIDS as a means of committing suicide. *American Journal of Psychiatry*, **142**, 656.

Frankl, D., Oye, R. K. & Bellamy, P. E. (1989). Attitudes of hospitalized patients toward life support: a survey of 200 medical inpatients. *American Journal of Medicine*, **86**, 645–8.

Franzblau, A., Letz, R., Hershman, D., Mason, P., Wallace, J. I. & Bekesi, J. G. (1991). Quantitative neurologic and neurobehavioral testing of persons infected with human immunodeficiency virus type 1. *Archives of Neurology*, **48**, 263–8.

Fraser, M. (1987). *Dementia. Its Nature and Management*. England: John Wiley.

Friedland, G. H., Saltzman, B. R., Rogers, M. F., Kahl, P. A., Lesser, M. L., Mayers, M. M. & Klein, R. S. (1986). Lack of transmission of HTLV-III/LAV infection to household contacts of patients with AIDS or AIDS-related complex with oral candidiasis. *New England Journal of Medicine*, **314**, 344–9.

Friedland, G..H. & Klein, R. S. (1987). Transmission of the human immunodeficiency virus. *New England Journal of Medicine*, **317**, 1125–35.

Friedman, S. R., Des Jarlais, D. C. & Sterk, C. E. (1990). AIDS and the social relations of intravenous drug users. *Millbank Quarterly*, **68**, 85–110.

Frost, D. P. (1985). Recognition of hypochondriasis in a clinic for sexually transmitted disease. *Genitourinary Medicine*, **61**, 133-?.

Funk, S. C. & Houston, B. K. (1987). A critical analysis of the Hardiness Scale's validity and utility. *Journal of Personal and Social Psychology*, **53**, 572–8.

Gala, C., Pergami, G. C., Catalan, J., Riccio, M., Durbano, F., Musicco, M., Baldeweg, T. & Invernizzi, G. (1992). Risk of deliberate self-harm and factors associated with suicidal behaviour among asymptomatic individuals with human immunodeficiency virus infection. *Acta Psychiatrica Scandinavica*, **86**, 70–5.

Gallagher, M., Foy, C., Rhodes, T., Philips, P., Setters, J., Moore, M., Naji, S., Donaldson, C. & Bond, J. (1990). HIV infection and AIDS in England and Wales: general practitioners' workload and contact with patients. *British Journal of General Practice*, **40**, 154–7.

Gary-Toft, P. & Anderson, J. G. (1981). Stress among hospital nursing staff: its causes and effects. *Social Science and Medicine*, **15**, 639–47.

Gattari, P., Spizzichion, L., Valenzi, C., Zaccarelli, M. & Rezza, G. (1992). Behavioural patterns and HIV infection among drug using transvestites practising prostitution in Rome. *AIDS Care*, **4**, 83–7.

Geddes, A. M. (1986). Risk of AIDS to health care workers. *British Medical Journal*, **292**, 711–12.

Gerbet, B., Maguire, B., Badner, B., Altman, D. & Stone, G. (1988). Why fear persists: health care professionals and AIDS. *Journal of the American Medical Association*, **260**, 3481–3.

Gibb, D. M., Duggan, C. & Lewin, R. (1991). The family and HIV. *Genito Urinary Medicine*, **67**, 363–6.

Gibbs, A., Andrews, D. G., Szmukler, G., Mulhall, B. & Bowden, S. C. (1990). Early HIV-related neuropsychological impairment: relationship to stage of viral infection. *Journal of Clinical and Experimental Neuropsychology*, **12**, 766–80.

Gillon, R. (1985). Confidentiality. *British Medical Journal*, **21**, 1634–66.

Gillon, R. (1987*a*). Refusal to treat AIDS and HIV positive patients. *British Medical Journal*, **294**, 1332–3.

Gillon, R. (1987*b*). AIDS and medical confidentiality. *British Medical Journal*, **294**, 1675–7.

Glanz, A. (1986*a*). Findings of a national survey of the role of general practitioners in the treatment of opiate misuse: dealing with the opiate misuser. *British Medical Journal*, **293**, 486–8.

Glanz, A. (1986*b*). Findings of a national survey of the role of general practitioners in the treatment of opiate misuse: views on treatment. *British Medical Journal*, **293**, 543–5.

Glanz, A. & Taylor, C. (1986). Findings of a national survey of the role of general practitioners in the treatment of opiate misuse: extent of contact with opiate misusers. *British Medical Journal*, **293**, 427–30.

Glass, R. M. (1988). AIDS and suicide. *Journal of the American Medical Association*, **259**, 1369–70.

Goethe, K. E., Mitchell, J. E., Marshall, D. W., Brey, R. L., Cahill, W. T., Leger, D., Hoy, L. J. & Boswell, R. N. (1989). Neuropsychological and neurological function of human immunodeficiency virus seropositive asymptomatic individuals. *Archives of Neurology*, **46**, 129–33.

Goffman, E. (1968). *Stigma*. Prentice-Hall.

Goldberg, D. P., Cooper, B., Eastwood, M. R., Kedward, H. B. & Shepherd, M. (1970). A standardised psychiatric interview for use in community studies *Journal of Preventive and Social Medicine*, **24**, 18–23.

Goldmeier, D. & Johnson, A. (1982). Does psychiatric illness affect the recurrence rate of genital herpes? *British Journal of Venereal Diseases*, **58**, 40–3.

Gorman, J. M. & Kertzner, R. (1990). Psychoneuroimmunology and HIV infection. *Journal of Neuropsychiatry and Clinical Neurosciences*, **2**, 241–52.

Gorman, J. M., Kertzner, R., Cooper, T., Goetz, R. R., Lagomasino, I., Novacenko, H., Williams, J. B. W., Stern, Y., Mayeux, R. & Ehrhardt, A. A. (1991). Glucocorticoid level and neuropsychiatric symptoms in homosexual men with HIV infection. *American Journal of Psychiatry*, **148**, 41–5.

Grant, I. & Atkinson, J. H. (1990). The evolution of neurobehavioural complications of HIV infection. *Psychological Medicine*, **20**, 747–54.

Grant, I., Atkinson, J. H., Hesselink, J. R., Kennedy, C. R., Richman, D. D., Spector, S. A. & McCutchen, J. A. (1987). Evidence for early central nervous system involvement in the acquired immunodeficiency syndrome (AIDS) and other human immunodeficiency virus (HIV) infections. *Annals of Internal Medicine*, **107**, 828–36.

Gravenor, D. S., Leclerc, J. R. & Blake, G. (1986). Tricyclic antidepressant agranulocytosis. *Canadian Journal of Psychiatry*, **31**, 661.

Gray, D. (1988). Counsellors in general practice. *Journal of the Royal College of General Practitioners*, **38**, 50–1.

Guy, P. J. (1987). AIDS: a doctor's duty. *British Medical Journal*, **294**, 445.

Halstead, S., Riccio, M., Harlow, P., Oretti, R. & Thompson, C. (1988). Psychosis associated with HIV infection. *British Journal of Psychiatry*, **153**, 618–23.

Hammond, D., Maw, R. D. & Mulholland, M. (1989). Personality types of women attending an STD clinic: correlation with keeping first review appointments. *Genitourinary Medicine*, **65**, 163–5.

Harding, T. W. (1987). AIDS in prison, *Lancet*, **ii**, 1260–4.

Harding, T. (1990). *HIV/AIDS in European Prisons*, WHO, Geneva.

Harris, M. J., Jeste, D. V., Gleghorn, A. & Sewell, D. (1991). New-onset psychosis in HIV-infected patients. *Journal of Clinical Psychiatry*, **52**, 369–76.

Hart, G., Fitzpatrick, R., McLean, J., Dawson, J. & Boulton, M. (1990). Gay men, social support and HIV disease: a study of social integration in the gay community. *AIDS Care*, **2**(2), 163–70.

Hart, G. J., Sonnex, C., Petherick, A., Johnson, A. M., Feinmann, C. & Adler, M. W. (1989). Risk behaviours for HIV infection among injecting drug users attending a drug dependency clinic. *British Medical Journal*, **298**, 1081–3.

Harter, D. H. (1989). Neuropsychological status of asymptomatic individuals seropositive to HIV-1. *Annals of Neurology*, **26**, 589–91.

Hausman, K. (1983). 'AIDS panic' brings lonely life to patients, gays. *Psychiatric News*, **August 19**, 3–25.

Henderson, A. S., Byrne, D. G. & Duncan-Jones, P. (1981). *Neurosis and the Social Environment*. Sydney: Academic Press.

Herns, M., Newman, S., McAllister, R., Weller, I. & Harrison, M. (1989). *Mood state, neuropsychology and self reported cognitive deficits in HIV infection*. Paper presented at the Vth International Conference on AIDS, Montreal.

Hickie, I., Silove, D., Hickie, C., Wakefield, D. & Lloyd, A. (1990). Is there immune dysfunction in depressive disorders? *Psychological Medicine*, **20**, 755–61.

Hintz, S., Kuck, J., Peterkin, J. J., Volk, D. M. & Zisook, S. (1990). Depression in the context of human immunodeficiency virus infection: implications for treatment. *Journal of Clinical Psychiatry*, **51**, 497–501.

Holland, J. C. & Tross, S. (1985). The psychosocial and neuropsychiatric sequelae of the acquired immunodeficiency syndrome and related disorders. *Annals of Internal Medicine*, **103**, 760–4.

Hooykaas, C., van der Linden, M. M. D., van Doornum, G. J. J., van der Velde, F. W., van der Pligt, J. & Coutinho, R. A. (1991). Limited changes in sexual behaviour of heterosexual men and women with multiple partners in the Netherlands. *AIDS Care*, **3**(1), 21–30.

Horstman, W. & McKusick, L. (1986). The impact of AIDS on the physician. In L. McKusick (Ed.), *What to do about AIDS* (pp. 63–74). Berkeley: University of California Press.

Hull, H. F., Mack Sewell, C., Wilson, J. & McFeeley, P. (1988). The risk of suicide in persons with AIDS. *Journal of the American Medical Association*, **260**(1), 29–30.

Hunt, A. J., Davies, P. M., Weatherburn, P., Coxon, A. P. M. & McManus, T. J. (1991). Changes in sexual behaviour in a large cohort of homosexual men in England and Wales,1988–9. *British Medical Journal*, **302**, 505–6.

Ikkos, G., Fitzpatrick, R., Frost, D. & Nazeer, S. (1987). Psychological disturbance and illness behaviour in a clinic for sexually transmitted diseases. *British Journal of Medical Psychology*, **60**, 121–6.

Irwin, M., Patterson, T., Smith, T. L., Caldwell, C., Borwn, S. A., Gillin, J. C. & Grant, I. (1990). Reduction of immune function in life stress and depression. *Biological Psychiatry*, **27**, 22–30.

Isomura, S. & Mizogami, M. (1992). The low rate of HIV infection in Japanese homosexual and bisexual men: an analysis of HIV seroprevalence and behavioural risk factors. *AIDS*, **6**, 501–3.

Jacob, K. S., John, J. K., Verghese, A., & John, T. J. (1987). AIDS-phobia. *British Journal of Psychiatry*, **150**, 412.

Jacoby, R. & Bergmann, K. (1991). Testamentory capacity. In R. Jacoby & C. Oppenheimer (Eds.), *Psychiatry in the Elderly* (pp. 924–927). Oxford: Oxford University Press.

Janssen, R. S., Saykin, A. J., Cannon, L., Campbell, J., Pinsky, P. F., Hessol, N. A., O'Malley, P. M., Lifson, A. R., Doll, L. S., Rutherford, G. W. & Kaplan, J. E. (1989). Neurological and neuropsychological manifestations of HIV-1 infection: association with AIDS-related complex but not asymptomatic HIV-1 infection. *Annals of Neurology*, **26**, 592–600.

Jenike, M. A. & Pato, C. (1986). Disabling fear of AIDS responsive to imipramine. *Psychosomatics*, **27**, 143–4.

Joffe, R. T., Rubinow, D. R., Squillace, K., Lane, C. H., Duncan, C. C. & Fauci, A. S. (1986). Neuropsychiatric aspects of AIDS. *Psychopharmacology Bulletin*, **22**, 684–8.

Johnson, A. M., Wadsworth, J., Elliott, P., Prior, L., Wallace, P., Blower, S., Webb, N. L., Heald, G. I., Miller, D. L., Adler, M. W. & Anderson, R. M. (1989). A pilot study of sexual lifestyle in a random sample of the population of Great Britain. *AIDS*, **3**, 135–41.

Johnstone, F. D., Brettle, R. P., MacCallum, L. R., Mok, J., Peutherer, F. & Burns, S. (1990). Women's knowledge of their HIV antibody state: its effect on their decision whether to continue the pregnancy. *British Medical Journal*, **300**, 23–4.

Johnstone, F. D., MacCullum, L., Brettle, R., Inglis, J. M. & Peutherer, J. F. (1988). Does infection with HIV affect the outcome of pregnancy? *British Medical Journal*, **296**, 467.

Joseph, J. G., Caumartin, S. M., Tal, M., Kirscht, J. P., Kessler, R. C., Ostrow, D. G. & Wortman, C. B. (1990). Psychological functioning in a cohort of gay men at risk for AIDS. *Journal of Nervous and Mental Disease*, **178**, 607–15.

Joseph, K. M., Adib, S. M., Joseph, J. G. & Tal, M. (1991). Gay identity and risky sexual behaviour related to the AIDS threat. *Journal of Community Health*, **16**, 287–97.

Kamenga, M., Ryder, R. W., Jingu, M., Mbuyi, N., Mbu, L., Behets, F., Brown, C. & Heyward, W. L. (1991). Evidence of marked sexual behaviour change associated with low HIV-1 seroconversion in 149 couples with discordant HIV-1 serostatus: experience at an HIV counselling center in Zaire. *AIDS*, **5**, 61–7.

Kaplan, H. B. (1989). Methodological problems in the study of psychosocial influences on the AIDS process. *Social Science and Medicine*, **29**, 277–92.

Kaplan, H. B. (1991). Social psychology of the immune system: a conceptual framework and review of the literature. *Social Science and Medicine*, **33**, 909–23.

Kaslow, R. A., Ostrow, D. G., Detels, R., Phair, J. P., Polk, B. F. & Rinaldo, C. R. (1987). The multicenter AIDS cohort study: rationale, organisation, and selected characteristics of the participants. *American Journal of Epidemiology*, **126**, 310–18.

Katoff, L., Rabkin, J. & Remien, R. H. (1991). *A psychological study of long term survivors of AIDS*. Paper presented at the VIIth International Conference on AIDS, Florence. Book of Abstracts Vol 1, TU. D.105.

Kavalier, F. C. (1989). Munchausen AIDS. *Lancet*, **i**, 852.

Kelly, J. A., St Lawrence, J. S., Smith, S., Hood, H. V. & Cook, D. J. (1987). Stigmatization of AIDS patients by their physicians. *American Journal of Public Health*, **77**, 789–91.

Kelly, J. A., St.Lawrence, J. S. & Brasfield, T. L. (1991). Predictors of vulnerability to AIDS risk behaviour relapse. *Journal of Consulting and Clinical Psychology*, **59**, 163–6.

Kelly, J. A., St.Lawrence, J. S., Diaz, Y. E., Stevenson, L. Y., Hauth, A. C., Brasfield, T. L., Kalichman, S. C., Smith, J. E. & Andrew, M. E. (1991). HIV risk behaviour reduction following intervention with key opinion leaders of population: an experimental analysis. *American Journal of Public Health*, **81**, 168–71.

Kelly, J. A., St.Lawrence, J. S., Hood, H. V. & Brasfield, T. L. (1989). Behavioural intervention to reduce AIDS risk activities. *Journal of Consulting and Clinical Psychology*, **57**, 60–7.

Kemeny, M. E., Duran, R., Taylor, S. E., Weiner, H., Visscher, B. & Fahey, J. L. (1990). *Chronic depression predicts CD4 decline over a five year period in HIV seropositive men*. Paper presented to the VIth International Conference on AIDS, San Francisco.

Kendler, K. S. (1986). A twin study of mortality in schizophrenia and neurosis. *Archives of General Psychiatry*, **43**, 643–9.

Kennedy, D. H., Nair, G., Elliott, L. & Ditton, J. (1991). Drug misuse and sharing of needles in Scottish prisons. *British Medical Journal*, **302**, 1507–8.

Kessler, R. C., Foster, C., Joseph, J., Ostrow, D., Wortman, C., Phair, J. & Chmiel, J. (1991). Stressful life events and symptom onset in HIV infection. *American Journal of Psychiatry*, **148**, 733–8.

Kieburtz, K., Zettelmaier, A. E., Ketonen, L., Tuite, M. & Caine, E. D. (1991). Manic syndrome in AIDS. *American Journal of Psychiatry*, **148**, 1068–70.

Kiely, B. G. & McPherson, I. G. (1986). Stress self-help packages in primary care: a controlled trial evaluation. *Journal of the Royal College of General Practitioners*, **36**, 307–9.

King, M. (1987). AIDS and the general practitioner: psycho-social issues. *Health Trends*, **19**, 1–3.

King, M. (1988). AIDS and the general practitioner: views of patients with HIV infection and AIDS. *British Medical Journal*, **297**, 182–4.

King, M. B. (1989*a*). Psychological and social problems in HIV infection: interviews with general practitioners in London. *British Medical Journal*, **299**, 713–17.

King, M. B. (1989*b*). Psychosocial status of 192 out-patients with HIV infection and AIDS. *British Journal of Psychiatry*, **154**, 237–42.

King, M. B. (1989*c*). AIDS on the death certificate: the final stigma. *British Medical Journal*, **298**, 734–6.

King, M. B. (1989*d*). London general practitioners: management of psychosocial problems in patients with HIV infection and AIDS. *Journal of the Royal College of General Practitioners*, **39**, 280–3.

King, M. B. (1992*a*). Male rape in institutional settings. In G. C. Mezey & M. B. King (Eds.), *Male Victims of Sexual Assault* (pp. 67–74). Oxford: Oxford University Press.

King, M. B. (1992*b*). Is there still a role for benzodiazepines in general practice? *British Journal of General Practice*, **42**, 202–5.

King's Fund Centre (1989). *Carers' needs: a ten point plan for carers' community care. Supplement for Carers for People*. London: King's Fund Centre.

Klee, H. (1991). *The potential for the sexual transmission of HIV: heroin and amphetamine injectors compared*. Paper presented to the VIIth International Conference on AIDS, Florence, Book of Abstracts Tu. D. 106.

Klee, H., Faugier, J., Hayes, C., Boulton, T. & Morris, J. (1990). AIDS-related risk behaviour, polydrug use and temazepam. *British Journal of Addiction*, **85**, 1125–32.

Klein, M. & Pfeffer, D. (1985). Homosexuality and the physician. *New Physician*, **September**, 43–8.

Kleyn, J. E., Day, L. E. & Weis, J. G. (1991). *Sex, lies and an alternative to videotapes: a comparison of monogamous sexual partners' self-reports*. Paper presented at the VIIth International Conference on AIDS, Florence. Book of Abstracts WC 3327.

Klimes, I., Catalan, J., Garrod, A., Day, A., Bond, A. & Rizza, C. (1992). Partners of men with HIV infection and haemophilia: controlled investigation of factors associated with psychological morbidity. *AIDS Care*, **4**, 149–56.

Kochen, M. M., Hasford, J. C., Jager, H., Zippel, S., L'age, M., Rosendahl, C., Fuebl, H. S. & Eichenlaub, D. (1991). How do patients with HIV perceive their general practitioners? *British Medical Journal*, **303**, 1365–8.

Koralink, I. J., Beaumanoir, A., Hausler, R., Kohler, A., Safran, A. B., Delacoux, R., Vibert, D., Mayer, E., Burkhard, P., Nahory, A., Magistris, M. R., Sanches, J., Myers, P., Paccolat, F., Quoex, F., Gabriel, V., Perrin, L., Mermillod, B., Gauthier, G., Waldvogel, F. A. & Hirschel, B. (1990). A controlled study of early neurologic abnormalities in men with asymptomatic human immunodeficiency virus infection. *New England Journal of Medicine*, **322**, 864–70.

Krahn, D. D., Nairn, K., Gosnell, B. A. & Drewnowski, A. (1991). *Journal of Clinical Psychiatry*, **52**, 112–15.

Kreiss, J., Carael, M. & Meheus, A. (1988). Role of sexually transmitted diseases in transmitting human immunodeficiency virus. *Genitourinary Medicine*, **64**, 1–2.

Lack, C. (1990). The 'I' becomes 'we'... then the 'we' becomes 'one'. A study of gay bereavement counselling. *Counselling*, **1**, 120–2.

Landesman, S. H., Minkoff, H. L. & Willoughby, A. (1989). HIV disease in reproductive age women: a problem of the present. *Journal of the American Medical Association*, **261**, 1326–7.

Lantos, P. L., McLaughlin, J. E., Scholtz, C. L., Berry, C. L. & Tighe, J. R. (1989). Neuropathology of the brain in HIV infection. *Lancet*, **i**, 309–11.

Lask, B. (1987). Forget the stiff upper lip. *British Medical Journal*, **295**, 1584–5.

Leach, G. & Whitehead, A. (1985). AIDS and the gay community: the doctor's role in counselling. *British Medical Journal*, **290**, 583.

Lee, C. A., Phillips, A. N., Elford, J., Janossy, G., Griffiths, P. & Kernoff, P. (1991). Progression of HIV disease in a haemophiliac cohort followed for 11 years and the effect of treatment. *British Medical Journal*, **303**, 1093–6.

Leigh, B. C. (1990). The relationship of sex-related alcohol expectancies to alcohol consumption and sexual behaviour. *British Journal of Addiction*, **85**, 919–28.

Lennon, M. C., Martin, J. L. & Dean, L. (1990). The influence of social support on AIDS-related grief reaction among gay men. *Social Science and Medicine*, **31**, 477–84.

Levine, C. (1990). AIDS and changing concepts of family. *Milbank Quarterly*, **68**, 33–58.

Levine, S. & Ursin, H. (1991). What is stress? In Brown, M. R., Koob, G. F. & Rivier, C. (eds) *Stress. Neurobiology and Neuroendocrinology* Marcel Dekker, New York.

Lewin, C. & Williams, R. J. W. (1988). Fear of AIDS: the impact of public anxiety in young people. *British Journal of Psychiatry*, **153**, 823–4.

Lewis, C. E., Freeman, H. E. & Corey, C. R. (1987). AIDS-related competence of California's primary care physicians. *American Journal of Public Health*, **77**, 795–9.

Lewis, C. E., Freeman, H. E., Kaplan, S. H. & Corey, C. R. (1986). The impact of a program to enhance the competencies of primary care physicians in caring for patients with AIDS. *Journal of General Internal Medicine*, **1**, 287–94.

Lifson, A. R., Hessol, N., Rutherford, G., O'Malley, P., Barnhart, L., Buchbinder, S., Cannon, L., Bodecker, T., Holmberg, S., Harrison, J. & Doll, L. (1990). *Natural history of HIV infection in a cohort of homosexual and bisexual men: clinical and immunologic outcome, 1977–1990*. Paper presented to the VIth International Conference on AIDS, San Francisco, Book of Abstracts Th. C. 33.

Link, R. N., Feingold, A. R., Charap, M. H., Freeman, K. & Shelov, S. P. (1988). Concerns of medical and pediatric house officers about acquiring AIDS from their patients. *American Journal of Public Health*, **78**, 455–9.

Linn, B. S., Linn, M. W. & Jenson, J. (1982). Degree of depression and immune responsiveness. *Psychosomatic Medicine*, **44**, 128–9.

Linn, B. S., Spiegel, J. S., Mathews, W. C., Leake, B., Lien, R. & Brooks, S. (1989). Recent sexual behaviours among homosexual men seeking primary medical care. *Archives of Internal Medicine*, **149**, 2685–90.

Ljungberg, B. & Christensson, B. (1991). *Still no HIV epidemic among local drug users at four year follow-up of the first Swedish syringe exchange program*. Paper presented to the VIIth International Conference on AIDS, Florence, Book of Abstracts WC 3290.

Logan, F. A., Maclean, A., Howie, C. A., Gibson, B., Hann, I. M. & Parry-Jones, W. L. (1990). Psychological disturbance in children with haemophilia. *British Medical Journal*, **301**, 1253–6.

Logsdail, S., Lovell, K., Warwick, H. & Marks, I. (1991). Behavioural teatment of AIDS-focused illness phobia. *British Journal of Psychiatry*, **159**, 422–5.

Lundy, S. (1989). HIV testing and mental disorder. *Journal of Medical Ethics*, **15**, 92–3.

Lunn, S., Skydsberg, M., Schulsinger, H., Parnas, J., Pedersen, C. & Mathiesen, L. (1991). A preliminary report on the neuropsychologic sequelae of human immunodeficiency virus. *Archives of General Psychiatry*, **48**, 139–42.

McArthur, J. C., Cohen, B. A., Selnes, O. A., Kumar, A. J., Cooper, K., McArthur, J. H., Soucy, G., Cornblath, D. R., Chmeil, J. S., Wang, M., Starkey, D. L., Ginzburg, H., Ostrow, D., Johnson, R. T., Phair, J. P. & Polk, B. F. (1989). Low prevalence of neurological and neuropsychological abnormalities in otherwise healthy HIV-1 infected individuals: results from the multicenter AIDS cohort study. *Annals of Neurology*, **26**, 601–11.

McArthur, J. C., Kumar, A. J., Johnson, D. W., Selnes, O. A., Becker, J. T., Herman, C., Cohen, B. A., Saah, A. & Multicenter AIDS Cohort Study, (1990). Incidental white matter hyperintensities on magnetic resonance imaging in HIV-1 infection. *Journal of Acquired Immune Deficiency Syndromes*, **3**, 252–9.

McCann, K. & Wadsworth, E. (1992). The role of informal carers in supporting gay men who have HIV related illness: what do they do and what are their needs? *AIDS Care*, **4**, 25–34.

McClure, M. O. & Schulz, T. F. (1989). Origin of HIV. *British Medical Journal*, **298**, 1267–8.

McCusker, J., Stoddard, A. M., McDonald, M., Zapka, J. G. & Mayer, K. H. (1992). Maintenance of behavioural change in a cohort of homosexually active men. *AIDS*, **6**, 861–8.

McEvoy, M., Porter, K., Mortimer, P., Simmons, N. & Shanson, D. (1987). Prospective study of clinical, laboratory and ancillary staff with accidental exposures to blood or body fluids from patients infected with HIV. *British Medical Journal*, **294**, 1595–7.

McKegney, F. P. & O'Dowd, M. A. (1992). Suicidality and HIV status. *American Journal of Psychiatry*, **149**, 396–8.

McKegney, F. P., O'Dowd, M. A., Feiner, C., Selwyn, P., Drucker, E. & Friedland, G. H. (1990). A prospective comparison of neuropsychiatric function in HIV-seropositive and seronegative methadone-maintained patients. *AIDS*, **4**, 565–9.

McMillan, A. (1988). HIV in prisons. *British Medical Journal*, **297**, 873–4.

Madden, A., Swinton, M. & Gunn, J. (1990). Women in prison and use of illicit drugs before arrest. *British Medical Journal*, **301**, 1133.

Madden, A., Swinton, M. & Gunn, J. (1991). Drug dependence in prisoners. *British Medical Journal*, **302**, 880.

Magana, J. R. (1991). Sex, drugs and HIV: an ethnographic approach. *Social Science and Medicine*, **33**, 5–9.

Mahorney, S. L. & Cavenar, J. O. (1988). A new and timely delusion: the complaint of having AIDS. *American Journal of Psychiatry*, **145**, 1130–2.

Maj, M. (1990). Psychiatric aspects of HIV-1 infection and AIDS. *Psychological Medicine*, **20**, 547–63.

Maj, M., Janssen, R., Satz, P., Zaudig, M., Starace, F., Boor, D., Sughondhabirom, B., Bing, E. G., Luabeya, M. K., Ndetei, D., Riedel, R., Schulte, G. & Sartorius, N. (1991). The World Health Organisation's cross-cultural study on neuropsychiatric aspects of infection with the human immunodeficiency virus 1 (HIV-1). *British Journal of Psychiatry*, **159**, 351–6.

Mann, J. M., Quinn, T. C., Francis, H., Nzilambi, N., Bosenge, N., Bila, K., McCormick, J. B., Ruti, K., Asila, P. K. & Curran, J. W. (1986). Prevalance of HTLV-III/LAV in household contacts of patients with confirmed AIDS and controls in Kinshasa, Zaire. *Journal of the American Medical Society*, **256**, 721–4.

Mansfield, S. & Singh, S. (1989). The general practitioner and human immunodeficiency virus infection: an insight into patients' attitudes. *Journal of the Royal College of General Practitioners*, **39**, 104–5.

Martin, G. S., Serpelloni, G., Galvan, U., Rizzetto, A., Gomma, M., Morgante, S.

& Rezza, G. (1990). Behavioural change in injecting drug users: evaluation of an HIV/AIDS education programme. *AIDS Care*, **2**, 275–9.

Martin, J. L. (1988). Psychological consequences of AIDS-related bereavement among gay men. *Journal of Consulting and Clinical Psychology*, **56**, 856–62.

Marzuk, P. M., Tierney, H., Tardiff, K., Gross, E. M., Morgan, E. B., Hsu, M. & Mann, J. (1988). Increased risk of suicide in persons with AIDS. *Journal of the American Medical Association*, **259**, 1333–7.

Maslach, C. (1982). *Burnout – The Cost of Caring*. Englewood Cliffs, Prentice-Hall.

Maslach, C. & Jackson, S. (1981). The measurement of experienced burnout. *Journal of Occupational Behaviour*, **2**, 99–113.

Mayou, R. (1987). Burnout. *British Medical Journal*, **295**, 284–5.

Mellers, J, Smith, J. R., Harris J. R. W. & King M. B. (1991). *Case control study of psychosocial status in HIV seropositive women*. Paper presented at the VIIth International Conference on AIDS, Florence, Book of Abstracts MB2100.

Meystre-Agustoni, G., Hausser, D., Zimmerman, E. & Dubois-Arber, F. (1990). *Physicians as agents in the prevention of the HIV epidemic*. Paper presented at the VIIth International Conference on AIDS, Florence, Book of Abstracts WD 4019.

Miller, D., Acton, T. M. G. & Hedge, B. (1988). The worried well: their identification and management. *Journal of the Royal College of Physicians of London*, **22**, 158–65.

Miller, D. & Green, J. (1985). Psychological support and counselling for patients with acquired immune deficiency syndrome (AIDS). *Genito Urinary Medicine*, **61**, 273–8.

Miller, D., Green, J., Farmer, R. & Carroll, G. (1985). A 'pseudo-AIDS' syndrome following from fear of AIDS. *British Journal of Psychiatry*, **146**, 550–1.

Miller, D. & Riccio, M. (1990). Non-organic psychiatric and psychosocial syndromes associated with HIV-1 infection and disease. *AIDS*, **4**, 381–8.

Miller, E. N., Satz, P. & Visscher, B. (1991). Computerized and conventional neuropsychological assessment of HIV-1-infected homosexual men. *Neurology*, **41**, 1608–16.

Miller, R. & Bor, R. (1988). *AIDS A Guide to Clinical Counselling* London, Science Press.

Miller, R., Goldman, E., Bor, R. & Kernoff, P. (1989a). AIDS and children: some of the issues in haemophilia care and how to address them. *AIDS Care*, **1**, 59–65.

Miller, R., Goldman, E., Bor, R. & Kernoff, P. (1989b). Counselling children and adults about AIDS·HIV: the ripple effect on haemophilia care settings. *Counselling Psychology Quarterly*, **2**, 65–72.

Miller, R. & Harrington, C. (1989). HIV and haemophilia. *AIDS Care*, **1**, 212–15.

Milne, R. I. G. & Keen, S. M. (1988). Are general practitioners ready to prevent the spread of HIV? *British Medical Journal*, **296**, 533–5.

Milner, G. L. (1989). Organic reaction in AIDS. *British Journal of Psychiatry*, **154**, 255–7.

Ministry of Health & Scottish Home and Health Department (1965). *Drug Addiction: The Second Report of the Interdepartmental Committee*, HMSO, London.

Mok, J. (1988). HIV infection in children. *Journal of the Royal College of General Practitioners*, **38**, 342–4.

Morris, M. (1991). American legislation on AIDS. *British Medical Journal*, **303**, 325–6.

Morriss, R., Schaerf, F., Brandt, J., McArthur, J. & Folstein, M. (1992). AIDS and multiple sclerosis: neural and mental features. *Acta Psychiatrica Scandinavica*, **85**, 331–6.

Morton, A. D. & McManus, I. C. (1986). Attitudes to knowledge about the acquired deficiency syndrome: lack of a correlation. *British Medical Journal*, **293**, 1212.

Moss, A. R. (1987). AIDS and intravenous drug use: the real heterosexual epidemic. *British Medical Journal*, **294**, 389–90.

Moulton, J. M., Stempel, R. R., Bacchetti, P., Temoshok, L. & Moss, A. R. (1991). Results of a one year longitudinal study of HIV antibody test notification from the San Francisco General Hospital cohort. *Journal of the Acquired Immune Deficiency Syndrome*, **4**, 787–94.

Murphy, T. F. (1988). Is AIDS a just punishment? *Journal of Medical Ethics*, **14**, 154–60.

Murray, R. M. (1976). Characteristics and prognosis of alcoholic doctors. *British Medical Journal*, **2**, 1537–9.

Myers, J. K., Weissman, M. M., Tischler, G. L., Holzer, C. E., Leaf, P. J., Orvaschel, H., Anthony, J. C., Boyd, J. A., Burke, J. D., Kramer, M. & Stoltzman, R. (1984). Six-month prevalence of psychiatric disorders in three communities. *Archives of General Psychiatry*, **41**, 959–67.

Naber, D., Perro, C., Schick, U., Schmauss, M., Erfurth, A., Bove, D., Goebel, F. D. & Hippius, H. (1990). Psychiatric symptoms and neuropsychological deficits in HIV infection. *Neuropsychopharmacology*, 745–55.

Naji, S. A., Russell, I. T., Foy, C. J. W., Gallagher, M., Rhodes, T. J. & Moore, M. P. (1989). HIV infection and Scottish general practice: workload and current practice. *Journal of the Royal College of General Practitioners*, **39**, 234–8.

Navia, B. A., Eun-Sook, C., Petito, C. K. & Price, R. W. (1986*a*). The AIDS dementia complex:II Neuropathology. *Annals of Neurology*, **19**, 525–35.

Navia, B. A., Jordan, B. D. & Price, R. W. (1986*b*). The AIDS dementia complex: I Clinical features. *Annals of Neurology*, **19**, 517–24.

Neaigus, A., Sufian, M., Friedman, S. R., Goldsmith, D. S., Stepherson, B., Mota, P., Pascal, J. & Des-Jarlais, D. C. (1990). Effects of outreach intervention on risk reduction among intravenous drug users. *AIDS Education and Prevention*, **2**, 253–71.

Nelson, H. E. & Willison, J. (1991). *The National Adult Reading Test – Test Manual*. England: NFER-Nelson.

Neville, R. G., McKellican, J. F. & Foster, J. (1988). Heroin users in general practice: ascertainment and features. *British Medical Journal*, **296**, 755–8.

Ngugi, E. N., Simonsen, J. N., Bosire, M., Ronald, A. R., Plummer, F. A., Cameron, D. W., Waiyaki, P. & Ndinya-Achola, J. O. (1988). Prevention of transmission of human immunodeficiency virus in Africa: effectiveness of condom promotion and health education among prostitutes. *Lancet*, **ii**, 887–90.

Norell, J. S. (1986). In aid of doctors suffering from complaints about AIDS. *British Medical Journal*, **293**, 1213–15.

Norman, S. E., Studd, J. & Johnson, M. (1990). HIV infection in women. *British Medical Journal*, **301**, 1231–2.

Norman, S. E., Chediak, A. D., Kiel, M. & Cohn, M. A. (1990). Sleep disturbances in HIV-infected homosexual men. *AIDS*, **4**, 775–781.

O'Dowd, M. A., Natali, C., Orr, D. & McKegney, F. P. (1991). Characteristics of patients attending an HIV-related psychiatric clinic. *Hospital and Community Psychiatry*, **42**, 615–19.

Oates, J. K. & Gomez, J. (1984). Venereophobia. *British Journal of Hospital Medicine*, **June**, 435–6.

Ochitill, H., Dilley, J. & Kohlwes, J. (1991). Psychotropic drug prescribing for hospitalized patients with acquired immunodeficiency syndrome. *American Journal of Medicine*, **90**, 601–5.

Ostrow, D. G., Monjan, A., Joseph, J., VanRaden, M., Fox, R., Kingsley, Dr.L., Dudley, J. & Phair, J. (1989). HIV-related symptoms and psychological functioning in a cohort of homosexual men. *American Journal of Psychiatry*, **146**, 737–42.

Padian, N. S. (1990). Sexual histories of heterosexual couples with one HIV-infected partner. *American Journal of Public Health*, **80**, 990–1.

Page, J. B., Lai, S., Chitwood, D. D., Klimas, N. G., Smith, P. C. & Fletcher, M. A. (1990). HTLV-I/II seropositivity and death from AIDS among HIV-I seropositive intravenous drug users. *Lancet*, **335**, 1439–41.

Paine, S. L. & Briggs, D. (1988). Knowledge and attitudes of Victorian medical practitioners in relation to the acquired immunodeficiency syndrome. *Medical Journal of Australia*, **148**, 221–5.

Parker, G. (1987). Are the lifetime prevalence estimates in the ECA study accurate? *Psychological Medicine*, **17**, 275–82.

Parkes, C. M. (1972). *Bereavement: Studies of Grief in Adult Life*. New York: International Universities Press.

Parkes, C. M. (1986). Care of the dying: the role of the psychiatrist. *British Journal of Hospital Medicine*, **October**, 250–5.

Pedder, J. R. & Goldberg, D. P. (1970). A survey by questionnaire of psychiatric disturbance in patients attending a venereal diseases clinic. *British Journal of Venereal Diseases*, **46**, 58–61.

Penkower, l., Dew, M. A., Kingsley, L., Becker, J. T., Satz, P., Schaerf, F. W. & Sheridan, K. (1991). Behavioural, health and psychosocial factors and risk for HIV infection among sexually active homosexual men: the Multicenter AIDS Cohort Study. *American Journal of Public Health*, **81**, 194–6.

Perdices, M. & Cooper, D. A. (1990). Neuropsychologic investigation of patients with AIDS and ARC. *Journal of Acquired Immune Deficiency Syndromes*, **3**, 555–64.

Perez, M. & Farrant, J. (1988). Immune reactions and mental disorders. *Psychological Medicine*, **18**, 11–13.

Perry, S., Belsky-Barr, D., Barr, W. B. & Jacobsberg, L. (1989). Neuropsychological function in physically asymptomatic HIV-seropositive men. *Journal of Neuropsychiatry*, **1**, 296–302.

Perry, S., Fishman, B., Jacobsberg, L. & Frances, A. (1992). Relationships over 1 year between lymphocyte subsets and psychosocial variables among adults with infection by human immunodeficiency virus. *Archives of General Psychiatry*, **49**, 396–401.

Perry, S., Fishman, B., Jacobsberg, L., Young, J. & Frances, A. (1991). Effectiveness of psychoeducational interventions in reducing emotional distress after human immunodeficiency virus antibody testing. *Archives of General Psychiatry*, **48**, 143–7.

Perry, S., Jacobsberg, L. & Fishman, B. (1990*a*). Suicidal ideation and HIV testing. *Journal of the American Medical Association*, **263**, 679–82.

Perry, S., Jacobsberg, L. B., Fishman, B., Frances, A., Bobo, J. & Jacobsberg, B. K. (1990*b*). Psychiatric diagnosis before serological testing for the human immunodeficiency virus. *American Journal of Psychiatry*, **147**, 89–93.

Perry, S., Jacobsberg, L. B., Fishman, B., Weiler, P. H., Gold, J. W. M. & Frances, A. J. (1990*c*). Psychological responses to serological testing for HIV. *AIDS*, **4**, 145–52.

Perry, S. W. (1990). Organic mental disorders caused by HIV: update on early diagnosis and treatment. *American Journal of Psychiatry*, **147**, 696–710.

Perry, S. W. & Tross, S. (1984). Psychiatric problems of AIDS inpatients at the New York Hospital: preliminary report. *Public Health Reports*, **99**, 200–5.

Pilowski, L. & O'Sullivan, G. (1989). Mental illness in doctors. *British Medical Journal*, **298**, 269–70.

Pinching, A. J. (1986). AIDS:dilemmas for the psychiatrist. *Lancet*, **i**, 496–497.

Polan, H. J., Hellerstein, D. & Amchin, J. (1985). Impact of AIDS-related cases on an inpatient therapeutic milieu. *Hospital and Community Psychiatry*, **36**, 173–6.

Pollak, M. & Schiltz, M. (1991). *Changing determinants of risk behaviour in the French gay community*. Paper presented at the VIIth International Conference on AIDS, Florence. Book of Abstracts TH. D.57.

Portegies, P., de Gans, J., Lange, J. M. A., Derix, M. M. A., Speelman, H., Bakker, M., Danner, S. A. & Goudsmit, J. (1989). Declining incidence of AIDS dementia complex after introduction of zidovudine treatment. *British Medical Journal*, **299**, 819–21.

Potterat, J. J., Phillips, L. & Muth, J. B. (1987). Lying to military physicians about risk factors for HIV infections. *Journal of the American Medical Association*, **257**, 1727.

Power, K. G., Markova, I., Rowlands, A., McKee, K. J., Anslow, P. J. & Kilfedder, C. (1991). Sexual behaviour in Scottish prisons. *British Medical Journal*, **302**, 1477–8.

Power, K. G., Markova, I., Rowlands, A., McKee, K. J., Anslow, P. J. & Kilfedder, C. (1992). Intravenous drug use and HIV transmission amongst inmates in Scottish prisons. *British Journal of Addiction*, **87**, 35–45.

Pradier, C., Carles, M., Durant, J., Bonifassi, L., Bernard, E., Mondain, V., DeSalvador, F. & Dellamonica, P. (1991). *Attitudes of general and specialists practitioners regarding HIV infection in southern France*. Paper presented to the VIIth International Conference on AIDS, Florence, Book of abstracts WD 4047.

Presidential Commission on the Human Innumodeficiency Virus Epidemic (1988). *Watkins Report*. Washington DC: United States Government Printing Office.

Price, R. W. & Brew, B. (1988). The AIDS dementia complex. *Journal of Infectious Diseases*, **158**, 1079–83.

Price, W. A. & Forejt, J. (1986). Neuropsychiatric aspects of AIDS: a case report. *General Hospital Psychiatry*, **8**, 7–10.

Prier, R. E., McNeil, J. G. & Burge, J. R. (1991). Inpatient Psychiatric Morbidity of HIV-infected soldiers. *Hospital and Community Psychiatry*, **42**, 619–23.

Prison Reform Trust (1988). *HIV, AIDS and Prisons*. London: Prison Reform Trust.

Rabkin, J. G. & Harrison, W. M. (1990). Effect of imipramine on depression and immune status in a sample of men with HIV infection. *American Journal of Psychiatry*, **147**, 495–7.

Rabkin, J. G., Williams, J. B. W., Neugebauer, R., Remien, R. H. & Goetz, R. (1990). Maintenance of hope in HIV-spectrum homosexual men. *American Journal Psychiatry*, **147**, 1322–6.

Rabkin, J. G., Williams, J. B. W., Remien, R. H., Goetz, R., Kertzner, R. & Gorman, J. M. (1991). Depression, distress, lymphocyte subsets, and human immunodeficiency virus symptoms on two occasions in HIV-positive homosexual men. *Archives of General Psychiatry*, **48**, 111–19.

Rajs, J. & Fugelstad, A. (1991). Suicide related to human immunodeficiency virus infection in Stockholm. *Acta Psychiatrica Scandinavica*, **85**, 234–9.

Rawnsley, K. (1986). Sick doctors. *Journal of the Royal Society of Medicine*, **79**, 440–1.

Raymond, C. A. (1988*a*). Lesbians call for greater physician awareness, sensitivity to improve patient care. *Journal of the American Medical Association*, **259**, 18.

Raymond, C. A. (1988*b*). Addressing homosexuals' mental health problems. *Journal of the American Medical Association*, **259**, 19.

Regier, D. A., Myers, J. K., Kramer, M., Robins, L. N., Blazer, D. G., Hough, R. L., Eaton, W. W. & Locke, B. Z. (1984). The NIMH epidemiological catchment area program. *Archives of General Psychiatry*, **41**, 934–41.

Reitan, R. M. & Wolfson, D. (1985). *The Halstead-Reitan Neuropsychological Test Battery: Theory and Clinical Interpretation*. Tucson, AZ: Neuropsychology Press.

Remien, R. H., Rabkin, J., Katoff, L. & Williams, J. (1991). *Suicidality and psychological outlook in long term survivors of AIDS*. Paper presented at the VIIth International Conference on AIDS, Florence. Book of Abstracts Vol 1, MD 105.

Rentoul, E. & Smith, H. (1973). *Glaisters Medical Jurisprudence and Toxicology*. London: Churchill-Livingstone.

Report of the Working Group of the American Academy of Neurology AIDS Task Force (1991). Nomenclature and research definitions for neurologic manifestations of human immunodeficiency virus-type 1 (HIV-1) infection. *Neurology*, **41**, 778–85.

Rey, A. (1964). *L'Examen Clinique en Psychologie*. Paris: Presses Universitaires de France.

Rhodes, T., Gallagher, M., Foy, C., Philips, P. & Bond, J. (1989). Prevention in practice: obstacles and opportunities. *AIDS Care*, **1**, 257–67.

Riccio, M., Pugh, K., Catalan, J., Jadresic, D., Baldweg, T. & Hawkins, D. (1991). *Neuropsychological findings in CDC group II gay men – one year follow-up of the St Stephen's cohort study*. Paper presented at the VIIth International Conference on AIDS, Florence, Book of Abstracts MB 2058.

Richards, T. (1988). Drug addicts and the GP. *British Medical Journal*, **296**, 1082.

Richardson, J. L., Lochner, T., McGuigan, K. & Levine, A. M. (1987). Physician attitudes and experience regarding the care of patients with acquired immunodeficiency syndrome (AIDS) and related disorders (ARC). *Medical Care*, **25**, 675–85.

Richings, J. C., Khara, G. S. & McDowell, M. (1986). Suicide in young doctors. *British Journal of Psychiatry*, **149**, 475–478.

Riedel, R.-R., Helmstaedter, C., Bulau, P., Durwen, H. F., Brackmann, H., Fimmers, R., Clarenbach, P., Miller, E. N. & Bottcher, M. (1991). Early signs of cognitive deficits among human immunodeficiency virus-positive haemophiliacs. *Acta Psychiatrica Scandinavica*, **85**, 321–6.

Roberts, J. J. K., Skidmore, C. A. & Robertson, J. R. (1989). Human immunodeficiency virus in drug misusers and increased consultation in general practice. *Journal of the Royal College of General Practitioners*, **39**, 373–4.

Robins, L. N., Helzer, J. E., Weissman, M. M., Orvaschel, H., Gruenberg, E., Burke, J. D. & Regier, D. A. (1984). Lifetime prevalence of specific psychiatric disorders in three sites. *Archives of General Psychiatry*, **41**, 949–58.

Roderick, P., Victor, C. R. & Beardow, R. (1990). Developing care in the community: GPs and the HIV epidemic. *AIDS Care*, **2**, 127–32.

Rose, K. D. & Rosow, I. (1973). Physicians who kill themselves. *Archives of General Psychiatry*, **29**, 800–5.

Rosendaal, F. R., Smit, C., Varekamp, I., Brocker-Vriends, A. H., van Dijck, H., Suurmeijer, T. P., Vandenbroucke, J. P. & Briet, E. A. D. (1990). Modern haemophilia treatment: medical improvements and quality of life. *Journal of International Medicine*, **228**, 633–40.

Ross, M. W. (1987). Illness behaviour among patients attending a sexually transmitted disease clinic. *Sexually Transmitted Diseases*, **14**, 174–9.

Ross, M. W. (1990). Reasons for non-use of condoms by homosexually active men during anal intercourse. *International Journal of Sexually Transmitted Diseases and AIDS*, **1**, 432–4.

Ross, M. W. (1992). Psychological determinants of increased condom use and safer sex in homosexual men: a longitudinal study. *International Journal of Sexually Transmitted Diseases and AIDS*, **1**, 98–101.

Ross, M. W., Gold, J., Wodak, A. & Miller, M. E. (1991). Sexually transmitted diseases in injecting drug users. *Genitourinary Medicine*, **67**, 32–6.

Ross, M. W. & Hunter, C. E. (1991). Dimensions, content and validation of the fear of AIDS schedule in health professionals. *AIDS Care*, **3**, 175–80.

Ross, M. W. & Seeger, V. (1988). Determinants of reported burnout in health professionals associated with the care of patients with AIDS. *AIDS*, **2**, 395–7.

Rosse, R. B. (1985). Reactions of psychiatric staff to an AIDS patient. *American Journal of Psychiatry*, **142**, 523.

Rowland, N. (1989). Can general practitioners counsel? *Journal of the Royal College of General Practitioners*, **39**, 435.

Rowland, N. & Irving, J. (1984). Towards a rationalisation of counselling in general practice. *Journal of the Royal College of General Practitioners*, **34**, 685–7.

Royal College of Nursing Working Party on AIDS (1986). *Nursing guidelines on the management of patients in hospital and the community suffering from AIDS*. London: Royal College of Nursing.

Royal, W., Updike, M., Selnes, O. A., Proctor, T. V., Nance-Sproson, L., Solomon, L., Vlahov, D., Cornblath, D. R. & McArthur, J. C. (1991). HIV-1 infection and nervous system abnormalities among a cohort of intravenous drug users. *Neurology*, **41**, 1905–10.

Rucinski, J. & Cybulska, E. (1985). Mentally ill doctors. *British Journal of Hospital Medicine*, **33**, 90–4.

Sacks, M., Dermatis, H., Looser-Ott, S., Burton, W. & Perry, S. (1992). Undetected HIV infection among acutely ill psychiatric inpatients. *American Journal of Psychiatry*, **149**, 544–5.

Salt, H., Miller, R. & Perry, L. (1989). Paradoxical interventions in counselling patients with intractable AIDS worry. *AIDS Care*, **1**, 39–44.

Sanders, S. C. (1984). Testamentory capacity. In J. G. Grimley-Evans & F. I. Caird (Eds.), *Advanced Geriatric Medicine* London: Pitman.

Schaerf, F. W., Miller, R. R., Lipsey, J. R. & McPherson, R. W. (1989). ECT for major depression in four patients infected with human immunodeficiency virus. *American Journal of Psychiatry*, **146**, 782–784.

Schafer, M. & Boyer, C. B. (1991). Psychosocial and behavioural factors associated with risk of sexually transmitted diseases, including human immunodeficiency virus infection, among urban high school students. *Journal of Pediatrics*, **119**, 826–33.

Schleifer, S. J., Keller, S. E., Bond, R. N., Cohen, J. & Stein, M. (1989). Major depressive disorder and immunity. *Archives of General Psychiatry*, **46**, 81–8.

Schmitt, F. A., Bigley, J. W. (1988). Neuropsychological outcome of zidovudine (AZT) treatment of patients with AIDS and AIDS-related complex. *New England Journal of Medicine*, **319**, 1573–8.

Scott, R. T. A. (1987). Attitudes towards patients infected with HIV. *Journal of the Royal College of General Practitioners*, **37**, 529–30.

Searle, E. S. (1987). Knowledge, attitudes and behaviour of health professionals in relation to AIDS. *Lancet*, **i**, 26–8.

Seeley, J., Wagner, U., Mulemwa, J., Kengeya-Kayondo, J. & Mulder, D. (1991). The development of a community-based HIV/AIDS counselling service in a rural area in Uganda. *AIDS Care*, **3**, 207–17.

Selwyn, P. A., Carter, R. J., Schoenbaum, E. E., Robertson, V. J., Klein, R. S. & Rogers, M. F. (1989). Knowledge of HIV antibody status and decisions to continue or terminate pregnancy among intravenous drug abusers. *Journal of the American Medical Association*, **261**, 3567–71.

Selzer, J. A. & Prince, R. (1985). Milieu complications of the psychiatric inpatient treatment of the AIDS patient. *Psychiatric Quarterly*, **57**, 77–80.

Seth, R., Granville-Grossman, K., Goldmeier, D. & Lynch, S. (1991). Psychiatric illness in patients with HIV infection and AIDS referred to the liaison psychiatrist. *British Journal of Psychiatry*, **159**, 347–50.

Shapiro, J. A. (1989). General practitioners' attitudes towards AIDS and their perceived information needs. *British Medical Journal*, **298**, 1563–6.

Shaw, G. M., Harper, G. M., Hahn, B. H., Epsterin, L. G., Gajdurisek, D. C., Price, R. W., Navia, B. A., Petito, C. K., O'Hara, C. J., Groopman, J. E., Cho, E. S., Oleske, J. M., Wong-Stall, F. & Gallo, R. C. (1985). HLTV-III infection in brains of children and adults. *Science*, **227**, 177–82.

Shearer, P. & McKusick, L. (1986). Counseling survivors. In McKusick, L. (ed). *What to do about AIDS* Berkeley, University of California Press, pp. 163–169.

Shelp, E. E., DuBose, E. R. & Sunderland, R. H. (1990). The infrastructure of religious communities: a neglected resource for care of people with AIDS. *American Journal of Public Health*, **80**, 970–2.

Sherr, L. (1991). *HIV and AIDS in Mothers and Babies*. Oxford: Blackwell.

Sherr, L. & Strong, C. (1992). Safe sex and women. *Genitourinary Medicine*, **68**, 32–5.

Shilts, R. (1987). *And The Band Played On*. New York: St Martin's Press.

Sibbald, B. & Freeling, P. (1988). AIDS and the future general practitioner. *Journal of the Royal College of General Practitioners*, **38**, 500–2.

Sibbald, B., Freeling, P., Coles, H. & Wilkins, J. (1991). HIV/AIDS workshop for primary health care staff. *Medical Education*, **25**, 243–50.

Siditis, J. J., Thaler, H., Brew, B. J., Sdaler, A. E., Keilp, J. G., Aranow, H. A. & Price, R. W. (1989). *The interval between equivocal and definite neurological symptoms in the AIDS dementia complex (ADC)*. Paper presented to the Vth International Conference on AIDS, Montreal.

Siegal, R. L. & Hoefer, D. D. (1981). Bereavement counselling for gay individuals. *American Journal of Psychotherapy*, **35**, 517–25.

Siegel, K., Mesagno, F. P., Chen, J. & Christ, G. (1989). Factors distinguishing homosexual males practising risky and safer sex. *Social Science and Medicine*, **28**, 561–9.

Smit, C., Rosendaal, F. & Varekamp, I. (1989). Physical condition, longevity and social importance of Dutch haemophiliacs, 1972–1985. *British Medical Journal*, **298**, 235–8.

Snider, W. D., Simpson, D. M., Nielsen, S., Gold, W. M., Metroka, C. E. & Posner, J. B. (1983). Neurological complications of acquired immune deficiency syndrome: analysis of 50 patients. *Annals of Neurology*, **14**, 403–18.

Sno, H. N., Storosum, J. G. & Swinkels, J. A. (1989). HIV infection: psychiatric findings in The Netherlands. *British Journal of Psychiatry*, **155**, 814–17.

Soloman, D. & Andrews, G. (eds). (1973). *Drugs and Sexuality* St Albans, Hertfordshire, Panther.

Spar, J. E. & Garb, A. S. (1992). Assessing competency to make a will. *American Journal of Psychiatry*, **149**, 169–74.

Spitzer, R., Williams, J. B., Gibbon, M. & First, M. (1988). *Structured Clinical Interview for DSMIIIR: Nonpatient version for HIV studies (SCID-NP-HIV* 6/1/88). New York: New York Psychiatric Institute.

Stall, R. D., Coates, T. J. & Hoff, C. (1988). Behavioural risk reduction for HIV infection among gay and bisexual men. *American Psychologist*, **43**, 878–85.

Steinbrook, R., Lo, B., Moulton, J., Saika, G., Hollander, M. H. & Volberding, P. A. (1986). Preferences of homosexual men with AIDS for life-sustaining treatment. *New England Journal of Medicine*, **314**, 457–60.

Stern, R. & Drummond, L. (1991). *The Practice of Behavioural and Cognitive Psychotherapy*. Cambridge: Cambridge University Press.

Stern, Y., Marder, K., Bell, K., Chen, J., Dooneief, G., Goldstein, S., Mindry, D., Richards, M., Sano, M., Williams, J., Gorman, J., Ehrhardt, A. & Mayeux, R. (1991). Multidisciplinary baseline assessment of homosexual men with and without human immunodeficiency virus infection. *Archives of General Psychiatry*, **48**, 131–8.

Stiffman, A. R., Dore, P., Earls, F. & Cunningham, R. (1992). The influence of mental health problems on AIDS-related risk behaviours in young adults. *Journal of Nervous and Mental Diseases*, **180**(5), 314–20.

Stimson, G. V. (1989). Syringe-exchange programmes for injecting drug users. *AIDS*, **3**, 253–60.

Strang, J. (1991). Injecting drug misuse. *British Medical Journal*, **303**, 1043–6.

Strang, J., Griffiths, P., Powis, B. & Gossop, M. (1992). First use of heroin: changes in route of administration over time. *British Medical Journal*, **304**, 1222–3.

Temoshok, L. (1988). Psychoimmunology and AIDS. In Bridge, T. P., Mirsky, A. F. & Goodwin, F. K. (eds). *Psychological, Neuropyschiatric and Substance Abuse Aspects of AIDS* Raven Press, New York, pp. 187–197.

The European Collaborative Study (1988). Mother to child transmission of HIV infection. *Lancet*, **ii**, 1039–43.

Thomas, C. S., Toone, B. K., Komy, A., Harwin, B. & Farthing, C. P. (1985). HTLV-III and psychiatric disturbance. *Lancet*, **i**, 395–6.

Thompson, C., Isaacs, G., Supple, D. & Bercu, S. (1986). AIDS: dilemmas for the psychiatrist. *Lancet*, **i**, 269–70.

Tirelli, U., Rezza, G., Giuliani, M., Caprilli, F., Gentili, G., Lazzarin, A., Saracco, A. & De Mercato, R. (1989). HIV seroprevalence among 304 female prostitutes from four Italian towns. *AIDS*, **3**, 547–8.

Todd, J. (1989). AIDS as a current psychopathological theme. A report on five heterosexual patients. *British Journal of Psychiatry*, **154**, 253–5.

Tomlinson, D. R., Hillman, R. J., Harris, J. R. W. & Taylor-Robinson, D. (1991). Screening for sexually transmitted disease in London-based male prostitutes. *Genitourinary Medicine*, **67**, 103–6.

Treiber, F. A., Shaw, D. & Malcolm, R. (1987). Acquired immune deficiency syndrome: psychological impact on health personnel. *Journal of Nervous and Mental Disease*, **175**, 496–9.

Tross, S., Price, R. W., Navia, B., Thaler, H. T., Gold, J., Hirsch, D. A. & Siditis, J. J. (1991). Neuropsychological characterization of the AIDS dementia complex: a preliminary report. *AIDS*, **2**, 81–8.

Turner, S. (1992). Surviving sexual assault and sexual torture. In G. C. Mezey & M. B. King (Eds.), *Male Victims of Sexual Assault* (pp. 75–86). Oxford: Oxford University Press.

Vaillant, G. E., Sobowale, N. C. & McArthur, C. (1972). Some psychologic vulnerabilities of physicians. *New England Journal of Medicine*, **ii**, 372–5.

Valdiserri, E. V., Hartl, A. J. & Chambliss, C. A. (1988). Practices reported by incarcerated drug abusers to reduce risk of AIDS. *Hospital and Community Psychiatry*, **39**, 966–72.

Van den Boom, F. M. L. G., Mead, C., Gremmen, T. & Roozenburg, H. (1991). *AIDS, euthanasia and grief*. Paper presented at the VIIth International Conference on AIDS, Florence, Book of Abstracts, Vol 1, MD 55.

van den Hoek, J. A. R., van Haastrecht, H. J. A. & Coutinho, R. A. (1991). Homosexual prostitution among male drug users and its risk for HIV infection. *Genitourinary Medicine*, **67**, 303–6.

Van der Maas, P., Van Delden, J., Pijnenborg, L. & Looman, C. (1991). Euthanasia and other medical decisions concerning the end of life. *Lancet*, **338**, 669–74.

Van der Wal, G., Van Eijk, J., Leenen, H. J. J. & Spreeuwenberg, C. (1992*a*). Euthanasia and assisted suicide. I. How often is it practised by family doctors in the Netherlands? *Family Practice*, **9**, 130–4.

Van der Wal, G., Van Eijk, J., Leenen, H. J. J. & Spreeuwenberg, C. (1992*b*). Euthanasia and assisted suicide. II. Do Dutch family doctors act prudently? *Family Practice*, **9**, 135–40.

van Griensven, G. J. P., de Vroome, E. M. M., Goudsmit, J. & Coutinho, R. A. (1989). Changes in sexual behaviour and the fall in incidence of HIV infection among homosexual men. *British Medical Journal*, **298**, 218–21.

Viadro, C. I. & Earp, J. A. (1991). AIDS education and incarcerated women: a neglected opportunity. *Women-Health*, **17**, 105–17.

Vogel-Scibilia, S. E., Mulsant, B. H. & Keshavan, M. S. (1988). HIV infection presenting as psychosis: a critique. *Acta Psychiatrica Scandinavica*, **78**, 652–6.

Volberding, P. (1989). Supporting the health care team in caring for patients with AIDS. *Journal of the American Medical Association*, **261**, 747–8.

Vuorio, K. A., Aarela, E. & Lehtinen, V. (1990). Eight cases of patients with unfounded fear of AIDS. *International Journal of Psychiatry and Medicine*, **20**, 405–11.

Wadsworth, E. & McCann, K. (1992). Attitudes towards and use of general practitioner services among homosexual men with HIV infection or AIDS. *British Journal of General Practice*, **42**, 107–10.

Wallack, J. J. (1989). AIDS anxiety among health care professionals. *Hospital and Community Psychiatry*, **40**, 507–10.

Wallston, B. S., Alagna, S. W., DeVellis, B. M. & DeVellis, R. F. (1983). Social support and physical health. *Health Psychology*, **2**, 367–91.

Waring, E. M. (1974). Psychiatric illness in physicians: a review. *Comprehensive Psychiatry*, **15**, 519–30.

Webb, T., Schilling, R., Jacobson, B. & Babb, P. (1988). *Health at Work. A Report on Health Promotion at the Workplace* Health Education Authority, Research Report No. 22, London.

Wight, D. (1992). Impediments to safer heterosexual sex: a review of research with young people. *AIDS Care*, **4**(1), 11–23.

Wilkie, F. L., Eisdorfer, C., Morgan, R., Loewenstein, D. L. & Szapocznik, J. (1991). Cognition in early human immunodefiency virus infection. *Archives of Neurology*, **47**, 433–40.

Wilkins, J. W., Robertson, K. R., Snyder, C. R., Robertson, W. K., van der Horst, C. & Hall, C. D. (1991). Implications of self-reported cognitive and motor dysfunction in HIV-positive patients. *American Journal of Psychiatry*, **148**, 641–3.

Wilkinson, G. (1984). Psychotherapy in the market place. *Psychological Medicine* **14**, 23–6.

Williams, J. B. W., Rabkin, J. G., Remien, R. H., Gorman, J. M. & Ehrhardt, A. A. (1991). Multidisciplinary baseline assessment of homosexual men with and without human immunodeficiency virus infection. *Archives of General Psychiatry*, **48**, 124–30.

Willoughby, B. C., Schechter, M. T., Craib, K. G. B., Sestak, P., Montaner, J. S. G., Voigt, R., Maynard, M., Woodfall, B. & O'Shaughnessy, M. V. (1991). *Characteristics of risk takers among seronegative men in a gay cohort*. Paper presented at the VIIth International Conference on AIDS, Florence, Book of Abstracts WC 3003.

Wilson, D., Chiropo, P., Lavelle, S. & Mutero, C. (1989). Sex worker, client sex behaviour and condom use in Harare, Zimbabwe. *AIDS Care*, **1**, 269–80.

Wing, J. K. (1974). *Measurement and Classification of Psychiatric Symptoms* Oxford University Press.

Wing, J. K., Cooper, J. E. & Sartorius, N. (1974). *The Measurement and Classification of Psychiatric Symptoms*. London: Cambridge University Press.

Wong, M. C., Suite, N. D. A. & Labar, D. R. (1990). Seizures in human immunodeficiency virus infection. *Archives of Neurology*, **47**, 640–2.

Woodward, J. (1981). The diagnosis and treatment of psychosomatic vulvovaginitis. *Practitioner*, **225**, 1673–7.

Working Party of the Royal College of General Practitioners (1988). Human immunodeficiency virus infection and the acquired immune deficiency syndrome in general practice. *Journal of the Royal College of General Practitioners*, **38**, 219–25.

World Health Organisation (1990). *Global Program on AIDS*; *Report on the Second Consultation on the Neuropsychiatric Aspects of HIV-1 Infection. Reference Number WHO/GPA/MNH/*90.1. Geneva: WHO.

Worth, D. (1990). Women at high risk of HIV infection. In D. G. Ostrow (Ed.), *Behavioural Aspects of AIDS* (pp. 101–119). New York: Plenum.

Wu, A. W., Kennedy, C. J. & Paradise, M. (1988). Factitious false-positive test for HIV. *Journal of the American Medical Association*, **259**, 1647.

Zich, J. & Temoshok, L. (1987). Perceptions of social support in men with AIDS and ARC: relationships with distress and hardiness. *Journal of Applied Social Psychology*, **17**, 193–215.

Zuger, A. & O'Dowd, M. A. (1992). The baron has AIDS: a case of factitious human immunodeficiency virus infection and review. *Clinical Infectious Diseases*, **14**, 211–16.

INDEX